Diagnosing the Less Common Skin Tumors

Clinical Appearance and Dermoscopy Correlation

Diagnosing the Less Common Skin Tumors
Clinical Appearance and Dermoscopy Correlation

Edited by
Caterina Longo, MD, PhD
Associate Professor, Dermatology and Venereology
Università degli Studi di Modena e Reggio Emilia (UNIMORE)
Azienda Unità Sanitaria Locale – IRCCS di Reggio Emilia
Centro Oncologico ad Alta Tecnologia Diagnostica
Modena, Italy

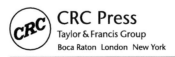

CRC Press is an imprint of the
Taylor & Francis Group, an **informa** business

CRC Press
Taylor & Francis Group
6000 Broken Sound Parkway NW, Suite 300
Boca Raton, FL 33487-2742

© 2019 by Taylor & Francis Group, LLC
CRC Press is an imprint of Taylor & Francis Group, an Informa business

No claim to original U.S. Government works

Printed on acid-free paper

International Standard Book Number-13: 978-1-138-10662-8 (Hardback)

This book contains information obtained from authentic and highly regarded sources. While all reasonable efforts have been made to publish reliable data and information, neither the author[s] nor the publisher can accept any legal responsibility or liability for any errors or omissions that may be made. The publishers wish to make clear that any views or opinions expressed in this book by individual editors, authors or contributors are personal to them and do not necessarily reflect the views/opinions of the publishers. The information or guidance contained in this book is intended for use by medical, scientific or health-care professionals and is provided strictly as a supplement to the medical or other professional's own judgement, their knowledge of the patient's medical history, relevant manufacturer's instructions and the appropriate best practice guidelines. Because of the rapid advances in medical science, any information or advice on dosages, procedures or diagnoses should be independently verified. The reader is strongly urged to consult the relevant national drug formulary and the drug companies' and device or material manufacturers' printed instructions, and their websites, before administering or utilizing any of the drugs, devices or materials mentioned in this book. This book does not indicate whether a particular treatment is appropriate or suitable for a particular individual. Ultimately it is the sole responsibility of the medical professional to make his or her own professional judgements, so as to advise and treat patients appropriately. The authors and publishers have also attempted to trace the copyright holders of all material reproduced in this publication and apologize to copyright holders if permission to publish in this form has not been obtained. If any copyright material has not been acknowledged please write and let us know so we may rectify in any future reprint.

Except as permitted under U.S. Copyright Law, no part of this book may be reprinted, reproduced, transmitted, or utilized in any form by any electronic, mechanical, or other means, now known or hereafter invented, including photocopying, microfilming, and recording, or in any information storage or retrieval system, without written permission from the publishers.

For permission to photocopy or use material electronically from this work, please access www.copyright.com (http://www.copyright.com/) or contact the Copyright Clearance Center, Inc. (CCC), 222 Rosewood Drive, Danvers, MA 01923, 978-750-8400. CCC is a not-for-profit organization that provides licenses and registration for a variety of users. For organizations that have been granted a photocopy license by the CCC, a separate system of payment has been arranged.

Trademark Notice: Product or corporate names may be trademarks or registered trademarks, and are used only for identification and explanation without intent to infringe.

Library of Congress Cataloging-in-Publication Data

Names: Longo, Caterina, MD, editor.
Title: Diagnosing the less common skin tumors : clinical appearance and dermoscopy correlation / edited by Caterina Longo.
Description: Boca Raton : CRC Press, [2019] | Includes bibliographical references and index.
Identifiers: LCCN 2019004947| ISBN 9781138106628 (hardback : alk. paper) | ISBN 9781315100555 (eBook)
Subjects: | MESH: Skin Neoplasms--diagnosis | Neoplasms, Glandular and Epithelial-- diagnosis | Dermoscopy--methods
Classification: LCC RC280.S5 | NLM WR 500 | DDC 616.99/477--dc23
LC record available at https://lccn.loc.gov/2019004947

Visit the Taylor & Francis Web site at
http://www.taylorandfrancis.com

and the CRC Press Web site at
http://www.crcpress.com

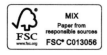

Printed and bound in Great Britain by
TJ International Ltd, Padstow, Cornwall

Contents

Contributors xi

SECTION I   Tumors of the Epidermis   1

1   Nevoid basal cell carcinoma syndrome   3
Stefania Borsari
Dermoscopy   4
References   5

2   Fibroepithelioma of Pinkus   7
Stefania Borsari
Dermoscopy   7
References   8

3   Basosquamous carcinoma   11
Stefania Borsari
Dermoscopy   12
References   13

4   Verrucous carcinoma   15
Stefania Borsari
Dermoscopy   16
References   17

5   Sarcomatoid squamous cell carcinoma   19
Stefania Borsari
Dermoscopy   20
References   20

SECTION II   Lentigines, Nevi, and Melanoma   23

6   Atypical Spitz nevus (tumor)   25
Caterina Bombonato
Introduction   25
Dermoscopy   25
References   27

7	**Halo Spitz nevus**	29
	Caterina Bombonato	
	Introduction	29
	Dermoscopy	30
	References	30
8	**Desmoplastic nevus**	31
	Caterina Bombonato	
	Introduction	31
	Dermoscopy	32
	References	32
9	**Pigmented epithelioid melanocytoma**	35
	Eugenia Veronica Di Brizzi, Gerardo Ferrara, Giuseppe Argenziano, and Elvira Moscarella	
	Introduction	35
	Dermoscopy	37
	References	37
10	**Animal-type melanoma**	39
	Caterina Bombonato	
	Introduction	39
	Dermoscopy	40
	References	40
11	**Nevoid melanoma**	43
	Caterina Bombonato	
	Introduction	43
	Dermoscopy	43
	References	44
12	**Balloon cell melanoma**	47
	Caterina Bombonato	
	Introduction	47
	Dermoscopy	47
	References	48
13	**Desmoplastic melanoma**	49
	Caterina Bombonato	
	Introduction	49
	Dermoscopy	50
	References	51
14	**Special site melanoma (mucosal, acral)**	53
	Caterina Bombonato	
	Introduction	53
	Dermoscopy	55
	References	56

SECTION III   Tumors of Cutaneous Appendages   59

15 Trichoadenoma   61
Riccardo Pampena
Introduction   61
Dermoscopy   62
References   62

16 Trichoepithelioma   63
Riccardo Pampena
Introduction   63
Dermoscopy   63
References   65

17 Desmoplastic trichoepithelioma   67
Riccardo Pampena
Introduction   67
Dermoscopy   68
References   68

18 Trichoblastoma   69
Riccardo Pampena
Introduction   69
Dermoscopy   70
References   71

19 Tumors of the follicular infundibulum   73
Riccardo Pampena
Introduction   73
Dermoscopy   73
References   74

20 Tricholemmoma and tricholemmal carcinoma and Cowden syndrome   77
Eugenia Veronica Di Brizzi, Simonetta Piana, Giuseppe Argenziano, and Elvira Moscarella
Introduction   77
Dermoscopy   78
References   79

21 Pilomatrixoma   81
Riccardo Pampena
Introduction   81
Dermoscopy   83
References   83

22 Fibrofolliculoma/trichodiscoma and Birt–Hogg–Dubè syndrome   85
Giovanni Paolino and Elvira Moscarella
Introduction   85
Dermoscopy   86
References   86

23 Sebaceous tumors — 89
Riccardo Pampena
Introduction — 89
Dermoscopy — 89
References — 91

24 Syringocystadenoma papilliferum — 93
Mara Lombardi
Introduction — 93
Dermoscopy — 94
References — 95

25 Hidradenoma — 97
Riccardo Pampena
Introduction — 97
Dermoscopy — 98
References — 99

26 Cylindroma and familial cylindromatosis and Brooke–Spiegler syndrome — 101
Riccardo Pampena
Introduction — 101
Dermoscopy — 101
References — 104

27 Spiradenoma — 105
Riccardo Pampena
Introduction — 105
Dermoscopy — 105
References — 106

28 Mammary and extramammary Paget's disease — 107
Riccardo Pampena, Giorgio La Viola, and Alessandro Annetta
Introduction — 107
Dermoscopy — 107
References — 109

29 Syringoma — 111
Riccardo Pampena
Introduction — 111
Dermoscopy — 112
References — 113

30 Eccrine poroma and eccrine porocarcinoma — 115
Riccardo Pampena
Introduction — 115
Dermoscopy — 115
References — 118

SECTION IV Mesenchymal Tumors   121

31 Dermatofibrosarcoma protuberans   123
Elisa Benati
Introduction   123
Dermoscopy   124
References   125

32 Atypical fibroxanthoma   127
Elisa Benati
Introduction   127
Dermoscopy   127
References   129

33 Malignant fibrous histiocytoma (pleomorphic undifferentiated sarcoma)   131
Elisa Benati
Introduction   131
Dermoscopy   131
References   132

SECTION V Other Uncommon Tumors   133

34 Merkel cell carcinoma   135
Elisa Benati
Introduction   135
Dermoscopy   135
References   137

35 Kaposi's sarcoma   139
Elisa Benati
Introduction   139
Dermoscopy   139
References   142

36 Angiosarcoma   143
Elisa Benati
Introduction   143
Dermoscopy   144
References   146

37 Retiform hemangioendothelioma   147
Elisa Benati
Introduction   147
Dermoscopy   147
References   148

Index   149

Contributors

Alessandro Annetta, MD
Azienda USL Latina
Latina, Italy

Giuseppe Argenziano, MD
Dermatology Unit
University of Campania Luigi Vanvitelli
Naples, Italy

Elisa Benati, MD
Centro Oncologico ad Alta Tecnologia
  Diagnostica
Azienda Unità Sanitaria Locale – IRCCS
  di Reggio Emilia
Reggio Emilia, Italy

Caterina Bombonato, MD
Centro Oncologico ad Alta Tecnologia
  Diagnostica
Azienda Unità Sanitaria Locale – IRCCS
  di Reggio Emilia
Reggio Emilia, Italy

Stefania Borsari, MD
Centro Oncologico ad Alta Tecnologia
  Diagnostica
Azienda Unità Sanitaria Locale – IRCCS
  di Reggio Emilia
Reggio Emilia, Italy

Eugenia Veronica Di Brizzi, MD
Dermatology Unit
University of Campania Luigi Vanvitelli
Naples, Italy

Gerardo Ferrara, MD
Anatomic Pathology Unit
Hospital of Macerata
Macerata, Italy

Giorgio La Viola, MD
Sezione Provinciale LILT Latina
Latina, Italy

Mara Lombardi, MD
Centro Oncologico ad Alta Tecnologia
  Diagnostica
Azienda Unità Sanitaria Locale – IRCCS
  di Reggio Emilia
Reggio Emilia, Italy

Elvira Moscarella, MD
Dermatology Unit
University of Campania Luigi Vanvitelli
Naples, Italy

Riccardo Pampena, MD
Centro Oncologico ad Alta Tecnologia
  Diagnostica
Azienda Unità Sanitaria Locale – IRCCS
  di Reggio Emilia
Reggio Emilia, Italy

Giovanni Paolino, MD
Unit of Dermatology
San Raffaele Scientific Institute (IRCCS)
Milan, Italy

Simonetta Piana, MD
Pathology Unit
Azienda Unità Sanitaria Locale – IRCCS
  di Reggio Emilia
Reggio Emilia, Italy

SECTION I

Tumors of the Epidermis

1 Nevoid basal cell carcinoma syndrome

Stefania Borsari

Nevoid basal cell carcinoma syndrome (NBCCS), also known as Gorlin–Goltz syndrome (GS), is an inherited autosomal dominant condition with high penetrance and variable expressivity.[1] NBCCS is caused by a germline mutation of the gene *PTCH1* on chromosome 9q22.3–q31.[2]

It is characterized by a triad of clinical manifestations: multiple basal cell carcinomas (BCCs), odontogenic jaw keratocysts and bifid ribs.[1] Besides this classic triad described by Gorlin and Goltz, a wide spectrum of developmental defects and tumors can be variably found in patients affected by this syndrome: calcification of the falx cerebri, palmar and plantar pits, spine anomalies, relative macrocephaly, facial milia, frontal bossing, ocular hypertelorism, medulloblastoma, ovarian fibroma, cleft lip or palate and the development of mental abnormalities.[3–5]

The incidence of NBCCS in the general population varies between 1:57,000 and 1:164,000, with a male-to female ratio of 1:1.[6,7]

The diagnosis is made when a series of established major and minor criteria are present, and it should be confirmed by DNA analysis.[7,8]

The cutaneous manifestations of the syndrome are the presence of multiple BCCs and acral pits.

The finding of multiple BCCs in a young person should raise the suspicion of NBCCS. In addition to their early onset during life (they typically appear during puberty) and their high number, BCCs of the NBCCS are less related to sun exposure than ordinary BCCs in nonsyndromic patients. Exposure to radiation therapy may lead to thousands of BCCs in the radiation field.[9] Although NBCCS represents only 0.4% of all cases of BCCs, early diagnosis is important for appropriate genetic counseling, avoidance of radiation, and timely adoption of photoprotection.[9,10]

Both nonsyndromic and syndromic BCCs are more commonly observed in patients with lighter skin. While BCCs occur in over 90% of whites with NBCCS, only 38%–44% of African Americans develop these tumors.[7,11]

Clinically, these lesions appear as pearly, flesh-colored or pigmented smooth papules, pedunculated lesions, nodules or plaques, sometimes covered by small blood vessels (Figures 1.1 and 1.2).[12,13] They can vary in number from just a few up to thousands, ranging in size from 1 to 10 mm or more in diameter, and tend to appear in unusual sites, like non-sun-exposed areas, the eyelid or the upper lip.[3,4,14,15]

At histopathologic examination, BCC associated with NBCCS does not differ from BCC arising in nonsyndromic patients.[5] About 30% of GS cases have two or more types of BCC histopathologic patterns (morphea-like, solid, superficial, cystic, adenoid, fibroepithelial or pigmented).[9,16]

The differential clinical diagnosis for these tumors includes melanocytic nevi, seborrheic keratosis, acrochordons, hemangiomas or molluscum contagiosum (Figure 1.2).[3]

Acral pits are another hallmark of NBCCS. They are observed in almost 50% of patients and are more common on the hands than on the feet.[12] They appear as pale, flesh-colored, pink or red millimetric depressions (Figure 1.3), which are totally asymptomatic and persist from their onset throughout life. Palmar pits are considered, by some authors, precursor lesions for BCCs.[17,18]

Although sporadic BCCs are generally managed with excisional surgery, considering the number and the recurrent nature of these lesions

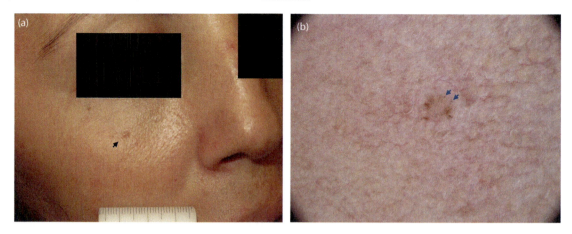

Figure 1.1 (a) A light brown smooth papule (arrow) on the right cheek of a 33-year-old woman affected by nevoid basal cell carcinoma syndrome. (b) In dermoscopy the lesion shows brown, black and some gray-blue dots (blue arrows), in the absence of additional specific BCC criteria (×20 original magnification).

in NBCCS, several alternative approaches have been proposed, including ablative laser therapy, electrocoagulation, cryosurgery, photodynamic therapy, topical imiquimod and 5-fluorouracil. The development of oral hedgehog pathway inhibitors has raised a new dimension to the current treatment of BCCs for patients affected by NBCCS.[19]

DERMOSCOPY

BCCs associated with NBCCS cannot be differentiated from those arising in nonsyndromic patients.[5] Then, BCCs in GS can be detected in early stages by the presence of typical, but often subtle, dermoscopic features of BCC.

BCCs in patients affected by NBCCS usually show arborizing vessels, ulceration and fine telangiectasias, in addition to blue-gray ovoid nests, dots and globules when pigmented.[20,21]

However, BCCs in these patients, especially when very small, may display a subtle dermoscopic aspect that makes diagnosis more difficult. Several authors, for example, described patients whose BCCs were typified only by dark brown and/or blue-gray dots or globules,

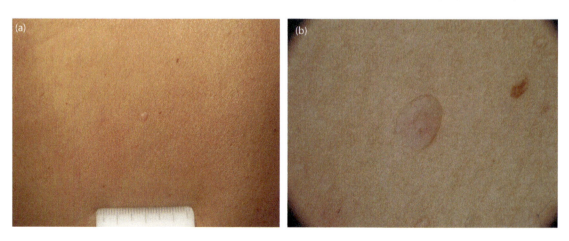

Figure 1.2 (a) The same patient presented, on her upper back, a translucent papule clinically resembling a dermal nevus. (b) The dermoscopic image of this papule shows arborizing vessels strongly suggestive for nodular BCC (×20 original magnification).

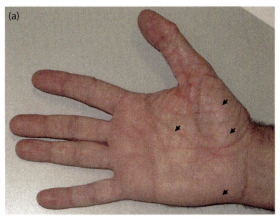 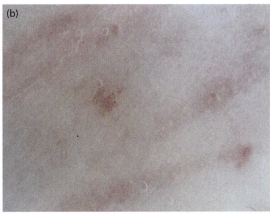

Figure 1.3 (a) The volar surface of the right hand of a 46-year-old man affected by NBCCS shows several white to red small depressions (arrows), known as "palmar pits." (b) On dermoscopy, the palmar pits show red globules regularly distributed in a linear fashion (×20 original magnification).

without any vascular pattern (Figure 1.1).[15,21–23] In longer-standing lesions, blue ovoid nests and arborizing vessels (Figure 1.2) are often observed. Also the presence of maple-leaf-like areas and spoke-wheel structures has been described.[15,21]

Acral pits show, on dermoscopy, small red or pink depressed lesions with sharp borders. Additional findings are red globules (Figure 1.3) that show a regular linear distribution, usually along the furrows.[21]

Jarrett and colleagues described two morphologically distinct types of pits: type 1 pits are composed of blue structures and microarborizing vessels and are more frequently seen in childhood; type 2 pits are characterized by a predominant vascular pattern of dotted vessels and are more frequently seen in adulthood.[24]

REFERENCES

1. Gorlin RJ, Goltz RW. Multiple nevoid basal cell epithelioma, jaw cysts and bifid rib: A syndrome. *N Engl J Med*. 1960;**262**:908–12.
2. Farndon PA, Del Mastro RG, Evans DG, Kilpatrick MW. Location of the gene for Gorlin syndrome. *Lancet*. 1992;**339**:581–2.
3. Gorlin RJ. Nevoid basal cell carcinoma syndrome. *Dermatol Clin*. 1995;**13**:113–25.
4. Manfredi M, Vescovi P, Bonanini M, Porter S. Nevoid basal cell carcinoma syndrome: A review of the literature. *Int J Oral Maxillofac Surg*. 2003;**33**:117–24.
5. Gutierrez MM, Mora RG. Nevoid basal cell carcinoma syndrome. A review and case report of a patient with unilateral basal cell nevus syndrome. *J Am Acad Dermatol*. 1986;**15**:1023–30.
6. Amezaga AOG, Arregui OG, Nuño SZ et al. Gorlin-Goltz syndrome: Clinicopathologic aspects. *Med Oral Patol Oral Cir Bucal*. 2008;**13**:338–43.
7. Kimonis VE, Goldstein AM, Pastakia B et al. Clinical manifestations in 105 persons with nevoid basal cell carcinoma syndrome. *Am J Med Genet*. 1997;**69**:299–308.
8. Evans DG, Ladusans EJ, Rimmer S et al. Complications of the naevoid basal cell carcinoma syndrome: Results of a population based study. *J Med Genet*. 1993;**30**:460–4.
9. Lo Muzio L. Nevoid basal cell carcinoma syndrome (Gorlin syndrome). *Orphanet J Rare Dis*. 2008;**3**:1–16.
10. Maddox WD, Winkelmann RK, Harrison EG et al. Multiple nevoid basal cell epitheliomas, jaw cysts and skeletal defects. *JAMA*. 1964;**188**:106–11.
11. Goldstein AM, Pastakia B, DiGiovanna JJ et al. Clinical findings in two African-American families with the nevoid basal cell carcinoma syndrome (NBCC). *Am J Med Genet*. 1994;**50**(3):272–81.
12. Gorlin RJ. Nevoid basal-cell carcinoma syndrome. *Medicine*. 1987;**66**:98–113.

13. Su CW, Lin KL, Hou JW et al. Spontaneous recovery from a medulloblastoma by a female with Gorlin-Goltz syndrome. *Pediatr Neurol.* 2003;**28**:231–4.
14. Honavar SG, Shields JA, Shields CL et al. Basal cell carcinoma of the eyelid associated with Gorlin-Goltz syndrome. *Ophthalmology.* 2001;**108**:1115–23.
15. Tiberio R, Valente G, Celasco M, Pertusi G, Veronese F, Bozzo C, Gattoni M, Colombo E. Pigmented basal cell carcinomas in Gorlin syndrome: Two cases with different dermatoscopic patterns. *Clin Exp Dermatol.* 2011;**36**:617–20.
16. Altamura D, Menzies SW, Argenziano G et al. Dermatoscopy of basal cell carcinoma: Morphologic variability of global and local features and accuracy of diagnosis. *J Am Acad Dermatol.* 2010;**62**:67–75.
17. Holubar K, Matras H, Smalik AV. Multiple palmar basal cell epitheliomas in basal cell nevus syndrome. *Arch Dermatol.* 1970;**101**:679.
18. Howell JB, Freeman RG. Structure and significance of the pits with their tumors in the nevoid basal cell carcinoma syndrome. *J Am Acad Dermatol.* 1980;**2**:224.
19. Ally MS, Tang JY, Joseph T et al. The use of vismodegib to shrink keratocystic odontogenic tumors in patients with basal cell nevus syndrome. *JAMA Dermatol.* 2014;**150**:542–5.
20. Tom WL, Hurley MY, Oliver DS et al. Features of basal cell carcinomas in basal cell nevus syndrome. *Am J Med Genet A.* 2011;**155A**:2098–104.
21. Kolm I, Puig S, Iranzo P et al. Dermoscopy in Gorlin-Goltz syndrome. *Dermatol Surg.* 2006;**32**:847–51.
22. Casari A, Argenziano G, Moscarella E, Lallas A, Longo C. Confocal and dermoscopic features of basal cell carcinoma in Gorlin-Goltz syndrome: A case report. *Australas J Dermatol.* 2017;**58**:e48–50.
23. Heck E, Kurwa H, Robertson L. Nevoid basal cell carcinomata mimicking melanocytic nevi: Case report. *J Cutan Med Surg.* 2018;**22**:349–52.
24. Jarrett R, Walker L, Bowling J. The dermoscopy of Gorlin syndrome: Pursuit of the pits revisited. *Arch Dermatol.* 2010;**146**:582–3.

2 Fibroepithelioma of Pinkus

Stefania Borsari

Fibroepithelioma of Pinkus (FeP) was first described in 1953 by Hermann Pinkus as a "premalignant fibroepithelial tumor of the skin."[1] He conceptualized FeP as a subtype of basal cell carcinoma (BCC), due to the histological finding of an anastomosing network of thin strands of basaloid cells embedded in a fibromatous stroma, arising from the undersurface of the epidermis and extending into the dermis. Although some authors consider it as a variant of trichoblastoma,[2,3] FeP has been definitively classified as a subtype of BCC, thanks to the use of a new immunostaining marker.[4]

FeP is relatively rare: in series of BCCs, its frequency ranges from 0.2% to 1.4%.[5–7] However, its real incidence is probably underestimated, since FeP may mimic a range of common benign skin tumors, such as dermal nevi, pedunculated fibromas, acrochorda and seborrheic keratoses, which are not usually excised or biopsied.

FeP has a predilection for females and is most commonly located on the lumbosacral region, although it may occur anywhere on the body surface, including extremities, chest/abdomen, head and genitalia (Figure 2.1).[7–10] It usually develops after the fourth decade of life, but a limited number of pediatric cases have also been described (Figure 2.2).[11,12] Typically, it is clinically seen as a solitary, rarely multiple, pink, flesh-colored or slightly brown-gray, well-demarcated sessile papule or plaque; large pedunculated, polypoid or ulcerated cases have also been reported.[8,13]

Being a variant of BCC, the best management includes early detection and complete surgical excision, which is considered curative.

DERMOSCOPY

To date, the dermoscopic features of only 26 FeP cases have been reported.[8,11,13–18] Of all published cases, 11 (42.3%) were pigmented; thus, pigmented FeP approaches one-half of all reported cases.

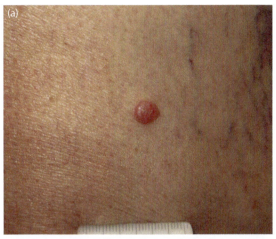

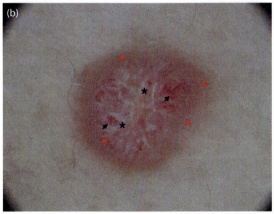

Figure 2.1 (a) A red, well-defined, smooth nodule on the right thigh of a 53-year-old woman. (b) On dermoscopy, the lesion shows, on a pinkish background, multiple white intersecting lines (asterisks) associated with fine, focused, short arborizing vessels (arrows) which become comma-like and dotted (red arrowheads) moving to the periphery of the lesion (×20 original magnification).

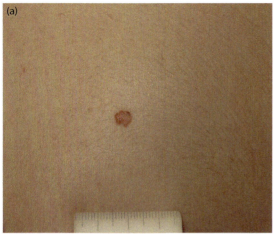
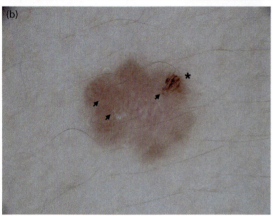

Figure 2.2 (a) One pink/light brown papule on the left scapular region of a 10-year-old girl; a little eccentric focus of hyperpigmentation is visible to the naked eye. (b) On dermoscopy, the lesion shows fine, focused, short linear and comma-like vessels on a variably pigmented background (from pink to light brown). Pigmented structures are visible at the periphery: small dark brown dots (arrows) and pigment network (asterisk) (×20 original magnification).

The dermoscopic characteristics of FeP, since the first case described in 2005,[14] have been well summarized by Reggiani et al.[8] as follows:

- Polymorphous vessels consisting mainly of fine, focused, short arborizing and dotted vessels (the latter mainly located at the periphery of the lesion), usually overlying a homogeneous white-pinkish coloration (Figures 2.1 and 2.2).
- Short white lines, also called chrysalis/crystalline structures, which appear as white septal lines throughout the tumor and are only visible when using polarized dermoscopy (Figure 2.1).
- Additional criteria, including milia-like cysts and erosions/ulceration, have been reported but are not specific for FeP.
- In case of pigmented FeP, gray-brown areas and gray-blue or brown dots can be seen (Figure 2.2).

REFERENCES

1. Pinkus H. Premalignant fibroepithelial tumors of skin. *Dermatol Syphilol*. 1953;**67**:598–615.
2. Hartschuh W, Schulz T. Merkel cell hyperplasia in chronic radiation-damaged skin: Its possible relationship to fibroepithelioma of Pinkus. *J Cutan Pathol*. 1997;**24**:477–83.
3. Bowen AR, LeBoit PE. Fibroepithelioma of Pinkus is a fenestrated trichoblastoma. *Am J Dermatopathol*. 2005;**27**:149–54.
4. Sellhever K, Nelson P, Kutzner H. Fibroepithelioma of Pinkus is a true basal cell carcinoma developing in association with a newly identified tumour-specific type of epidermal hyperplasia. *Br J Dermatol*. 2012;**166**:88–97.
5. Betti R, Inselvini E, Carducci M, Crosti C. Age and site prevalence of histologic subtypes of basal cell carcinomas. *Int J Dermatol*. 1995;**34**:174–6.
6. Rahbari H, Mehregan AH. Basal cell epitheliomas in usual and unusual sites. *J Cutan Pathol*. 1979;**6**:425–31.
7. Misago N, Narisawa Y. Polypoid basal cell carcinoma on the perianal region: A case report and review of the literature. *J Dermatol*. 2004;**31**:51–5.
8. Reggiani C, Zalaudek I, Piana S, Longo C, Argenziano G, Lallas A, Pellacani G, Moscarella E. Fibroepithelioma of Pinkus: Case reports and review of the literature. *Dermatology*. 2013;**226**:207–11.
9. Cohen PR, Tschen JA. Fibroepithelioma of Pinkus presenting as a sessile thigh nodule. *Skinmed*. 2003;**2**:385–7.
10. Scherbenske JM, Kopeloff IH, Turiansky G, Sau P. A solitary nodule on the chest: Fibroepithelioma of Pinkus. *Arch Dermatol*. 1990;**126**:955, 958.
11. Scalvenzi M, Francia MG, Falleti J, Balato A. Basal cell carcinoma with fibroepithelioma-like

11. histology in a healthy child: Report and review of the literature. *Pediatr Dermatol.* 2008;**25**:359–63.
12. Pan Z, Huynh N, Sarma DP. Fibroepithelioma of Pinkus in a 9-year-old boy: A case report. *Cases J.* 2008;**1**:21.
13. Zalaudek I, Ferrara G, Broganelli P, Moscarella E, Mordente I, Giacomel J, Argenziano G. Dermoscopy patterns of fibroepithelioma of Pinkus. *Arch Dermatol.* 2006;**142**:1318–22.
14. Zalaudek I, Leinweber B, Ferrara G, Soyer HP, Ruocco E, Argenziano G. Dermoscopy of fibroepithelioma of Pinkus. *J Am Acad Dermatol.* 2005;**52**:168–9.
15. Longo C, Soyer HP, Pepe P, Casari A, Wurm EM, Guitera P, Pellacani G. In vivo confocal microscopic pattern of fibroepithelioma of Pinkus. *Arch Dermatol.* 2012;**148**:556.
16. Viera M, Amini S, Huo R, Oliviero M, Bassalo S, Rabinovitz H. A new look at fibroepithelioma of Pinkus: Features at confocal microscopy. *J Clin Aesthet Dermatol.* 2008;**1**:42–4.
17. Roldán-Marín R, Ramírez-Hobak L, González-de-Cossio AC, Toussaint-Caire S. Fibroepithelioma of Pinkus in continuity with a pigmented nodular basal cell carcinoma (BCC): A dermoscopic and histologic correlation. *J Am Acad Dermatol.* 2016;**74**(5):e91–3.
18. Inskip M, Longo C, Haddad A. Two adjacent individual fibroepithelioma of Pinkus of the umbilicus—One pink, one pigmented—A case report and review of the literature. *Dermatol Pract Concept.* 2016;**6**:17–20.

3 Basosquamous carcinoma

Stefania Borsari

Basosquamous carcinoma was first described in the early twentieth century as a tumor with a histomorphology intermediate between basal cell carcinoma (BCC) and squamous cell carcinoma (SCC).[1] Later, a similar morphologic subtype of BCC was described, the metatypical BCC.[2] Over time, the terminology became confusing with some authors separating basosquamous from metatypical carcinoma, others using the terms synonymously and still others claiming the basosquamous carcinoma as a keratotic variant of BCC.[3–5]

Today, the basosquamous carcinoma is considered by most dermatologists a subtype of BCC with aggressive behavior and higher tendency for recurrence and metastases.

Retrospective studies suggest that this neoplasm represents from 1.2% to 2.7% of all BCCs.[6–8]

Basically, basosquamous carcinoma is a nonpigmented papule, plaque or nodule, with a "rust-red" color, ulceration and a history of rapid and/or aggressive growth (Figures 3.1 through 3.3).[5,6,8–12] However, its clinical appearance is considered nonspecific, as it can mimic a number of benign and malignant skin lesions, such as viral wart, seborrheic keratosis, hyperkeratotic actinic keratosis, Bowen's disease, BCC, invasive SCC and melanoma. For this reason, its recognition is difficult, and the diagnosis is often made only after a biopsy.

It occurs predominantly in men after the fifth decade of life. It is usually located on the head and neck (80% of cases), but it can also occur on the trunk and extremities.[5–13]

At histopathologic examination, this tumor shows areas of both classical BCC and SCC, with a transition zone between them. It has an infiltrative pattern with tongues of tumor cells embedded in a dense fibroblast-rich stroma.[6,7,14] With immunohistochemical stains, the areas of BCC are Ber-EP4,

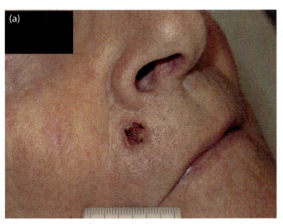 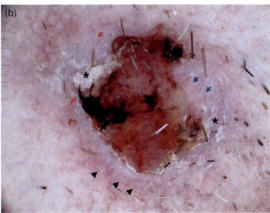

Figure 3.1 (a) An ulcerated plaque on the subnasal area of an 80-year-old man. This clinical aspect, with a raised peripheral border, suggests a BCC. (b) On dermoscopy, in addition to the large central blood crust, superficial scales (asterisks) and white circles (triangles) are visible. The vascular pattern is made by focused (blue arrows) and unfocused (red arrows) linear serpiginous vessels (×20 original magnification).

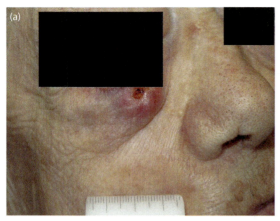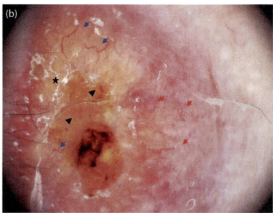

Figure 3.2 (a) A retracting, yellow/pink plaque of the lower eyelid in a 95-year-old patient. A central focus of ulceration is visible. (b) On dermoscopy, the lesion shows, beyond ulcerations, masses of keratin with blood spots within them (triangles), scales (asterisk) and both focused (blue arrows) and unfocused (red arrows) arborizing vessels at the periphery of the lesion (×20 original magnification).

AE1 and AE3 positive, whereas the areas of SCC are AE1, AE3 and CAM5.2 positive and show variable staining with epithelial membrane antigen.[15]

Basosquamous carcinoma has a worse prognosis and a greater risk of recurrence and metastases as compared to BCC. Its behavior can be equaled to that of SCC, so it seems logical to treat basosquamous carcinoma according to protocols followed for SCC.[5,13,14,16–18] Actually, the rate of distant metastasis of basosquamous carcinoma has been reported to be higher than for either BCC or SCC alone.[10]

Complete surgical removal is mandatory to avoid significant morbidity and even mortality related to this aggressive skin malignancy. Mohs micrographic surgery could be indicated for high-risk locations or recurrent or large tumors. Radiation is a good alternative in selected cases.

DERMOSCOPY

There are only two studies evaluating the dermoscopic features of basosquamous carcinoma, which analyzed 22 and 36 lesions, respectively.[19,20]

The dermoscopic appearance of basosquamous carcinoma reflects its peculiar histopathology, since it is characterized by features of both BCC and SCC.

The basosquamous carcinoma usually shows ulceration (blood crusts) and unfocused arborizing vessels, alone or in combination with dotted, linear, coiled, looped and/or focused arborizing vessels, preferentially located at the periphery of the tumor (Figures 3.1 and 3.2). A possible explanation for the unfocused appearance of vessels may be that they are visualized by dermoscopy through an acanthotic epidermis, in contrast to a thinned epidermis in classical BCC (which gives a focused appearance).

Blue-gray blotches (ovoid nests), another BCC-specific criterion, are quite common in basosquamous carcinoma (33%–59%), but similarly to arborizing vessels, they appear less well defined than in classical BCC (Figure 3.3). Of note, dermoscopy allows their detection even in a tumor with a nonpigmented clinical appearance.

Keratin masses (more or less centrally located, amorphous, yellow-white to light-brown areas that may contain reddish to red-black blood spots), whitish structureless areas, superficial scales, white structures, including white circles (targetoid hair follicles) and clods (keratin pearls) and blood spots in keratin masses, which are relatively frequent findings in invasive SCC or actinic keratosis, are also some

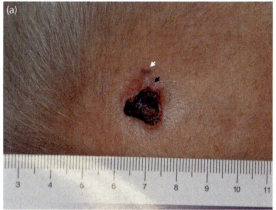 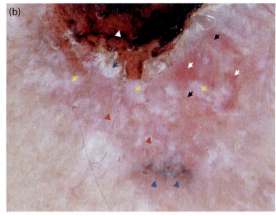

Figure 3.3 (a) An almost fully ulcerated lesion on the parieto-occipital region of an 85-year-old man. In the upper portion, there is a translucent pink area (black arrow) with a small eccentric focus of pigmentation (white arrow). (b) The dermoscopic image of the pink eccentric portion of the lesion is a good example of the coexistence, in basosquamous carcinoma, of BCC- and SCC-related dermoscopic criteria. BCC criteria are blue-gray dots and ovoid nests (blue triangles), focused arborizing vessels (red triangles) and ulceration (white triangle); SCC criteria are unfocused polymorphic vessels (black arrows) and red lacunae (white arrows), scales (blue arrow) and white structureless areas (yellow arrows) (×20 original magnification).

of the most common dermoscopic features observed in basosquamous carcinoma (Figures 3.1 through 3.3).

In the case series described by Giacomel et al.,[19] at least one BCC-like and one SCC-like dermoscopic characteristic are present in all but one basosquamous carcinomas (Figure 3.3). Hence, a simple practical suggestion is that the identification of at least one feature of both invasive SCC and BCC should raise suspicion for basosquamous carcinoma and lead to prompt definitive surgical removal.

REFERENCES

1. Hamilton M. Basal squamous cell epithelioma. *Arch Dermatol Syph*. 1928;**18**:50–73.
2. Strutton GM. Pathological variants of basal cell carcinoma. *Australas J Dermatol*. 1997;**38**(Suppl): S31–5.
3. Lennox B, Wells AL. Differentiation in the rodent ulcer group of tumors. *Br J Cancer*. 1951;**5**:195–212.
4. Elder DE, Elenitsas R, Johnson BL, Murphy GF. *Lever's histopathology of the skin*. 9th ed. Philadelphia, PA: Lippincott Williams & Wilkins, 2005.
5. Garcia C, Poletti E, Crowson AN. Basosquamous carcinoma. *J Am Acad Dermatol*. 2009;**60**(1):137–43.
6. Martin RC, Edwards MJ, Cawte TG, Sewell CL, McMasters KM. Basosquamous carcinoma: Analysis of prognostic factors influencing recurrence. *Cancer*. 2000;**88**:1365–9.
7. Schuller DE, Berg JW, Sherman G, Krause CJ. Cutaneous basosquamous carcinoma of the head and neck: A comparative analysis. *Otolaryngol Head Neck Surg*. 1979;**87**:420–7.
8. Bowman PH, Ratz JL, Knoepp TG, Barnes CJ, Finley EM. Basosquamous carcinoma. *Dermatol Surg*. 2003;**29**:830–2.
9. Betti R, Crosti C, Ghiozzi S et al. Basosquamous cell carcinoma: A survey of 76 patients and a comparative analysis of basal cell carcinomas and squamous cell carcinomas. *Eur J Dermatol*. 2013;**23**:83–6.
10. Mougel F, Kanitakis J, Faure M, Euvrard S. Basosquamous cell carcinoma in organ transplant patients: A clinicopathologic study. *J Am Acad Dermatol*. 2012;**66**:e151–7.
11. Boyd AS, Stasko TS, Tang YW. Basaloid squamous cell carcinoma of the skin. *J Am Acad Dermatol*. 2011;**64**:144–51.
12. Costantino D, Lowe L, Brown DL. Basosquamous carcinoma – An under-recognized, high-risk

cutaneous neoplasm: Case study and review of the literature. *J Plast Reconstr Aesthet Surg.* 2006;**59**:424–8.
13. Borel DM. Cutaneous basosquamous carcinoma. *Arch Pathol Lab Med.* 1973;**95**:293–7.
14. Lopes de Faria J, Nunes PH. Basosquamous cell carcinoma of the skin with metastases. *Histopathology.* 1988;**12**:85–94.
15. Jones MS, Helm KF, Maloney ME. The immunohistochemical characteristics of the basosquamous cell carcinoma. *Dermatol Surg.* 1997;**23**:181–4.
16. Maloney ML. What is basosquamous carcinoma? *Dermatol Surg.* 2000;**26**:505–6.
17. Barksdale SK, O'Connor N, Barnhill R. Prognostic factors for cutaneous squamous cell and basal cell carcinoma: Determinants of risk of recurrence, metastasis, and development of subsequent skin cancers. *Surg Oncol Clin N Am.* 1997;**6**:625–38.
18. Randle HW. Basal cell carcinoma: Identification and treatment of the high-risk patient. *Dermatol Surg.* 1996;**22**:255–61.
19. Giacomel J, Lallas A, Argenziano G, Reggiani C, Piana S, Apalla Z, Ferrara G, Moscarella E, Longo C, Zalaudek I. Dermoscopy of basosquamous carcinoma. *Br J Dermatol.* 2013;**169**(2):358–64.
20. Akay BN, Saral S, Heper AO, Erdem C, Rosendahl C. Basosquamous carcinoma: Dermoscopic clues to diagnosis. *J Dermatol.* 2017;**44**(2):127–34.

4 Verrucous carcinoma

Stefania Borsari

In 1948 Ackerman[1] described verrucous carcinoma (VC), a rare variant of well-differentiated, low-grade squamous cell carcinoma (SCC).

It is characterized by a low metastatic potential, but it can be locally aggressive (with invasion of soft tissues, muscles and bone) with a tendency to recur after excision. It is a slow-growing tumor, chronically evolving from a discrete focal lesion to a large deeply penetrating solitary mass.[2]

The three major locations of VC are the oral cavity (where it is also known as *oral florid papillomatosis*), the *anogenital region* (*giant condyloma of Buschke and Löwenstein*) and the palmoplantar surfaces (*epithelioma cuniculatum*).[3–5] More rare locations such as the buttock, sacral region and ear have also been described.[6,7]

It occurs predominantly in males in their fourth to seventh decades of life. It is usually associated with human papillomavirus (HPV) infection. Smoking, alcohol consumption, immunodeficiency, chronic inflammation or trauma, irradiation or arsenic ingestion are also considered inducing factors.[8–12]

In general, VC clinically appears as a papillary gray-white or red mass with a very broad base of attachment and measuring up to several centimeters. The name *verrucous* derives from the presence of epithelial projections and keratin-filled invaginations.

More specifically, oral VC usually appears as a large hyperkeratotic nodule mostly located in the alveolar mucosa, tongue or hard palate; although this is the most common site of occurrence, it has a low incidence, accounting for almost 5% of all oral carcinomas.[13]

Anogenital verrucous carcinoma clinically appears as a papillomatous gray-whitish plaque (Figure 4.1) or a cauliflower-like tumor.

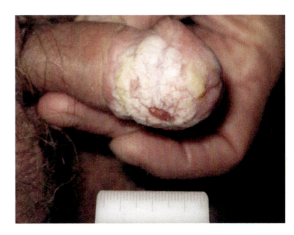

Figure 4.1 A genital verrucous carcinoma in a 67-year-old man with a history of genital warts. The tumor looks like a large plaque with a papillomatous white surface and few red foci of ulceration.

Palmoplantar VC occurs predominantly on the soles (Figure 4.2) and on the anterior weight-bearing areas, but can occur also on the palms (Figure 4.3). It usually appears as a fungating, exophytic mass with numerous keratin-filled sinuses. As the tumor grows, it locally invades soft tissues until reaching the plantar fascia and advances toward the dorsal surface of the foot, with destruction of the metatarsal bones occurring.[5,14] A history of a nonhealing wart on the soles, palms or other locations should raise suspicion of VC and lead the physician to perform a biopsy. A deep biopsy specimen of the lesion is necessary, as superficial portions may resemble a verruca vulgaris.

The differential diagnosis of VC includes verruca vulgaris, reactive epidermal hyperplasia, infundibular cyst, benign adnexal tumor, giant seborrheic keratosis, pyogenic granuloma, leukoplakia, eccrine poroma, hyperkeratotic basal

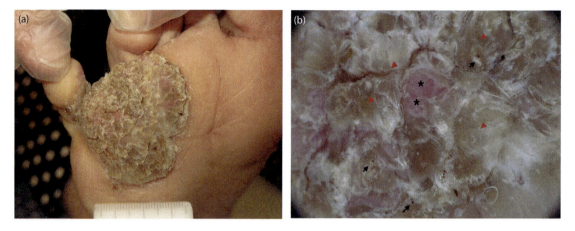

Figure 4.2 (a) A verrucous carcinoma on the right sole of a 51-year-old immunocompromised woman, appearing as a well-defined exophytic mass with numerous keratinic protuberances and invaginations. (b) On dermoscopic examination, the lesion shows numerous amorphous keratin masses (red triangles), red dotted and coiled vessels in papillary pink-whitish structures (asterisks), and black dots (black arrows) (×20 original magnification).

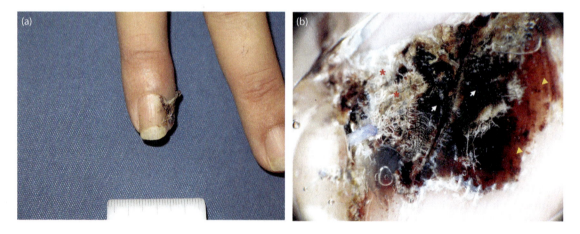

Figure 4.3 (a) A periungual verrucous carcinoma on the right hand of a 57-year-old man, appearing as a black-red-whitish-colored crusty lesion. In this case, dermoscopy is crucial to exclude the presence of clues suggestive of melanocytic lesion. (b) On dermoscopy, the lesion does not show criteria suggestive of melanocytic lesion, but does show blood crusts (white arrows), keratin (red asterisks) and subcorneal hemorrhages (yellow triangles) (×20 original magnification).

cell epithelioma, well-differentiated squamous cell carcinoma and melanoma.[3,14,15]

First-line treatment is wide local excision with a 5 mm margin of healthy tissue to avoid recurrence. In more severe cases, amputation of a toe or even a foot has been described. Electrodessication, cryotherapy and laser ablation often fail.[16]

DERMOSCOPY

To date, neither clinical studies nor report cases describing the dermoscopic aspects of VC have been published.

Our clinical experience suggests that there are no specific dermatoscopic clues useful to make an early diagnosis of VC. Just the clinical appearance and the evolution (progressive slow growth and resistance to treatments) should lead to suspicion of VC and lead the clinician to perform a deep biopsy.

Dermoscopy is definitely important for making a differential diagnosis with other malignant tumors, in particular acral melanoma. In the case of acral verrucous melanoma, the early detection of melanoma-specific dermatoscopic findings (such as pigmented parallel-ridge pattern) allows unpleasant diagnostic delays that would have important consequences for the patient to be avoided.[15,17]

Given the epithelial nature of these tumors and the high grade of differentiation, we could observe amorphous keratin structures and keratin masses.

REFERENCES

1. Ackerman LV. Verrucous carcinoma of the oral cavity. *Surgery*. 1948;**23**:670–8.
2. Spiro RH. Verrucous carcinoma, then and now. *Am J Surg*. 1998;**176**(5):393–7.
3. Ho J, Diven DG, Butler PJ, Tyring SK. An ulcerating verrucous plaque on the foot. *Arch Dermatol*. 2000;**136**:550–1.
4. Schein O, Orestein A, Bar-Meir E. Plantar verrucous carcinoma (epithelioma cuniculatum): Rare form of the commonest wart. *Isr Med Assoc J*. 2006;**8**(12):885.
5. Aird I, Johnson HD, Lennox B, Stansfeld AG. Epithelioma cuniculatum: A variety of squamous carcinoma peculiar to the foot. *Br J Surg*. 1954;**42**(173):245–50.
6. Costache M, Desa LT, Mitrache LE, Patrascu OM, Dumitru A, Costache D, Albu E, Sajin M, Simionescu O. Cutaneous verrucous carcinoma – Report of three cases with review of literature. *Rom J Morphol Embryol*. 2014;**55**:383–8.
7. Rinaldo A, Devaney KO, Ferlito A. Verrucous carcinoma of the ear: An uncommon and difficult lesion. *Acta Otolaryngol*. 2004;**124**(3):228–30.
8. Thavaraj S, Cobb A, Kalavrezos N, Beale T, Walker DM, Jay A. Carcinoma cuniculatum arising in the tongue. *Head Neck Pathol*. 2012;**6**:130–4.
9. Fonseca FP, Pontes HA, Pontes FS et al. Oral carcinoma cuniculatum: Two cases illustrative of a diagnostic challenge. *Oral Surg Oral Med Oral Pathol Oral Radiol* 2013;**116**:457–63.
10. Pons Y, Kerrary S, Cox A et al. Mandibular cuniculatum carcinoma: Apropos of 3 cases and literature review. *Head Neck*. 2012;**34**:291–5.
11. Allon D, Kaplan I, Manor R, Calderon S. Carcinoma cuniculatum of the jaw: A rare variant of oral carcinoma. *Oral Surg Oral Med Oral Pathol Oral Radiol Endod* 2002;**94**:601–8.
12. Raguse JD, Menneking H, Scholmann HJ, Bier J. Manifestation of carcinoma cuniculatum in the mandible. *Oral Oncol Extra*. 2006;**42**:173–5.
13. Depprich RA, Handschel JG, Fritzemeier CU, Engers R, Kübler NR. Hybrid verrucous carcinoma of the oral cavity: A challenge for the clinician and the pathologist. *Oral Oncol Extra*. 2006;**42**(2):85–90.
14. Kathuria S, Rieker J, Jablokow VR, Van den Broek H. Plantar verrucous carcinoma (epithelioma cuniculatum): Case report with review of the literature. *J Surg Oncol*. 1986;**31**(1):71–5.
15. Dalmau J, Abellaneda C, Puig S, Zaballos P, Malvehy J. Acral melanoma simulating warts: Dermoscopic clues to prevent missing a melanoma. *Dermatol Surg*. 2006;**32**(8):1072–8.
16. Zielonda E, Goldschmidt D, Fontaine S. Verrucous carcinoma or epithelioma cunuculatum plantae. *Eur J Surg Oncol*. 1997;**23**:86–7.
17. Argenziano G, Soyer HP, Chimenti S et al. Dermoscopy of pigmented skin lesions: Results of a consensus meeting via the Internet. *J Am Acad Dermatol*. 2003;**48**:679–93.

5 Sarcomatoid squamous cell carcinoma

Stefania Borsari

The spindle cell or sarcomatoid squamous cell carcinoma (SSCC) is an uncommon variant of squamous cell carcinoma (SCC). It is a high-grade, aggressive tumor with the possibility of local recurrence and lymph node or distant metastasis. It consists of an irregular growth of atypical spindle-shaped cells in the dermis: the atypical spindle cells may constitute all or part of the tumor, with none or a variable component of conventional SCC forming nests, cords and keratin pearls; the tumor often infiltrates deep into the dermis, subcutis, fascia, muscle and bone.[1-3]

It belongs to the group of *malignant cutaneous spindle cell tumors*, which also includes atypical fibroxanthoma, desmoplastic melanoma and leiomyosarcoma.

The differential diagnosis among these entities is quite easy when the lesion displays a more well-differentiated component or an in situ component; more commonly, their distinction relies on the expression of immunohistochemical-specific markers: in addition to cytokeratins, p63 is one of the most reliable markers for SSCC.[4-6]

SSCC tends to occur preferentially in men, on skin exposed to solar or ionizing radiation (mainly head and neck), and in patients older than 50 years.[7,8] Several cases that occurred on genitalia (penis) have been described in even younger patients.[9-13]

In the few published case reports, SSCC is described in its clinical appearance as a single, firm, ulcerated, brown-red or reddish-gray nodule, measuring 1 cm to a few centimeters in diameter (Figures 5.1 and 5.2).[10,14,15] This clinical presentation is unspecific and is compatible with a series of malignant cutaneous tumors, such as SCC, atypical fibroxanthoma, amelanotic melanoma and Merkel cell carcinoma. Faced with such a clinical aspect, a prompt, complete surgical excision is mandatory.

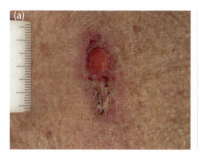
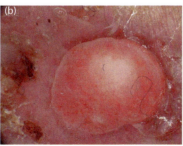
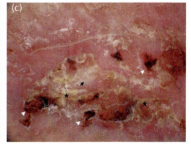

Figure 5.1 (a) A 61-year-old man presented a sarcomatoid squamous cell carcinoma (SSCC) on his neck appearing as a red nodule in the center of an eroded plaque covered with yellow-dark crusts. (b) The nodule, on dermoscopic examination, shows a reddish color and a surface covered by linear irregular vessels (×20 original magnification). (c) The flat, eroded portion shows blood crusts (white triangles), white structureless areas (black arrow) and yellow scales (asterisks) (×20 original magnification).

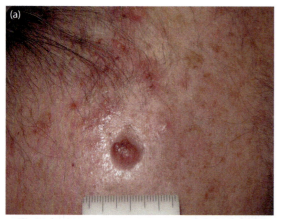

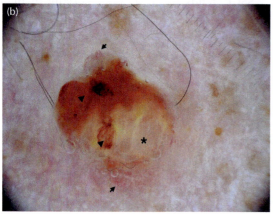

Figure 5.2 (a) An SSCC on the scalp of an 85-year-old man, clinically appearing as an opaque red nodule with a surface partially covered by yellow-reddish crusts. (b) On dermoscopy, this nodular lesion shows ulceration (triangles), white structureless areas (asterisk) and linear irregular vessels at the periphery (arrows) (×20 original magnification).

DERMOSCOPY

To date, only one case of SSCC has been described in its dermatoscopic appearance.[15] Omori et al. reported a case of a 67-year-old woman with a 6-month history of a hard, reddish-gray nodule on her left ear; dermoscopic examination detected a polymorphous vascular pattern made of dotted/glomerular and linear irregular vessels, white structureless areas, yellow to light-brown opaque scales and microerosions/ulcerations.

Our cases (Figures 5.1 and 5.2) look quite similar to those reported in the literature in their clinical and dermoscopic aspects: these are reddish nodular lesions that dermoscopically show linear irregular vessels, ulceration, white structureless areas and yellowish scales.

All dermoscopic features described, in the absence of white structures (like white circles or targetoid hair follicles with a predominant red color), are suggestive of a poorly differentiated SCC.[16,17] SSCC does not seem to have specific dermatoscopic features.

REFERENCES

1. Silvis NG, Swanson PE, Manivel JC et al. Spindle-cell and pleomorphic neoplasms of the skin. A clinicopathologic and immunohistochemical study of 30 cases, with emphasis on "atypical fibroxanthomas." *Am J Dermatopathol.* 1988;**10**(1):9–19.
2. Evans HL, Smith JL. Spindle cell squamous carcinomas and sarcoma-like tumors of the skin: A comparative study of 38 cases. *Cancer.* 1980;**45**(10):2687–97.
3. Martin HE, Stewart FW. Spindle cell epidermoid carcinoma. *Am J Cancer Res.* 1935;**24**(2):273–98.
4. Gleason BC, Calder KB, Cibull TL et al. Utility of p63 in the differential diagnosis of atypical fibroxanthoma and spindle cell squamous cell carcinoma. *J Cutan Pathol.* 2009;**36**:543.
5. Kanner WA, Brill LB 2nd, Patterson JW, Wick MR. CD10, p63 and CD99 expression in the differential diagnosis of atypical fibroxanthoma, spindle cell squamous cell carcinoma and desmoplastic melanoma. *J Cutan Pathol.* 2010;**37**:744.
6. Ha Lan TT, Chen SJ, Arps DP, Fullen DR, Patel RM, Siddiqui J, Carskadon S, Palanisamy N, Harms PW. Expression of the p40 isoform of p63 has high specificity for cutaneous sarcomatoid squamous cell carcinoma. *J Cutan Pathol.* 2014;**41**:831–8.
7. Cassarino DS, DeRienzo DP, Barr RJ. Cutaneous squamous cell carcinoma: A comprehensive clinicopathologic classification. *J Cutan Pathol.* 2006;**33**:261–79.
8. Chang NJ, Kao DS, Lee LY, Chang JW, Hou MM, Lam WL, Cheng MH. Sarcomatoid carcinoma in head and neck: A review of 30 years of experience—Clinical outcomes and reconstructive results. *Ann Plast Surg.* 2013;**71**:1–7.

9. Zhou M, Netto GJ, Epstein JI. Sarcomatoid (spindle cell) squamous cell carcinoma of the penis. In: Zhou M, ed. *Uropathology: High-yield pathology*. Philadelphia, PA: Elsevier; 2012:496–7.
10. Svitlana Y, Bachurska SY, Antonov PA, Staykov DG, Dechev IY. Sarcomatoid squamous cell carcinoma of the penis—A report of two cases. *Folia Medica*. 2017;59:232–7.
11. Velazquez EF, Melamed J, Barreto JE et al. Sarcomatoid carcinoma of the penis: A clinicopathologic study of 15 cases. *Am J Surg Pathol*. 2005;29:1152–8.
12. Lont AP, Gallee M, Snijders P et al. Sarcomatoid squamous cell carcinoma of the penis: A clinical and pathological study of 5 cases. *J Urol*. 2004;172:932–5.
13. Axcrona K, Brennhovd B, Andersen M et al. Sarcomatoid squamous cell carcinoma of the penis. *Act Onco*. 2010;49:128–30.
14. Kogame T, Tanimura H, Nakamaru S, Makimura K, Okamoto H, Kiyohara T. Spindle cell squamous cell carcinoma arising in Bowen's disease: Case report and review of the published work. *J Dermatol*. 2017;44:1055–8.
15. Omori Y, Nobeyama Y, Tomita S, Ishida K, Nakagawa H. Case of spindle cell squamous cell carcinoma with dermoscopic findings of diffuse/discrete scales and predominant white color. *J Dermatol*. 2016;43:1239–41.
16. Zalaudek I, Giacomel J, Schmid K et al. Dermatoscopy of facial actinic keratosis, intraepidermal carcinoma, and invasive squamous cell carcinoma: A progression model. *J Am Acad Dermatol*. 2012;66:589–97.
17. Lallas A, Pyne J, Kyrgidis A et al. The clinical and dermoscopic features of invasive cutaneous squamous cell carcinoma depend on the histopathological grade of differentiation. *Br J Dermatol*. 2015;172:1308–15.

SECTION II

Lentigines, Nevi, and Melanoma

6 Atypical Spitz nevus (tumor)

Caterina Bombonato

INTRODUCTION

Atypical Spitz tumors (ASTs) are defined as melanocytic proliferations with intermediate histopathologic features between Spitz nevi and Spitzoid melanoma, carrying uncertain malignant potential.[1–10]

In 1989, Smith and colleagues[2] described the "Spitz nevus with atypia and metastasis." A few years later, Barnhill et al.[3,4] defined the category of metastasizing Spitz tumor, or atypical Spitz tumor. Recently, these lesions have been included in the group of melanocytic tumors of uncertain malignant potential.[11,12] Currently there are three interpretations regarding the taxonomy of ASTs:

1. they are nevi that have features in common with melanoma but are biologically benign,
2. they are intermediates between nevi and melanomas,
3. they represent a subset of melanomas with a better prognosis than conventional melanomas.[13]

Clinically, ASTs are often more than 10 mm in diameter, with asymmetric shape, irregular borders, irregular or ulcerated surface and irregular distribution of colors (Figures 6.1 through 6.4).

The management of ASTs is not clearly defined. Some authors think surgical margins should be enlarged to at least 1 cm, and others recommend sentinel lymph node biopsy, even if a recent systematic review done by Lallas et al.[14] did not prove the utility of this procedure.

DERMOSCOPY

In the literature, few papers describe dermoscopic features of ASTs. Ferrara et al.[8] reported pediatric ASTs as large, nodular, fast-growing, sometimes ulcerated lesions, divided into "red"

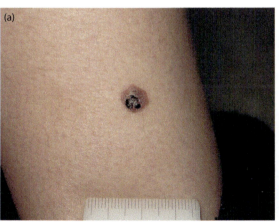 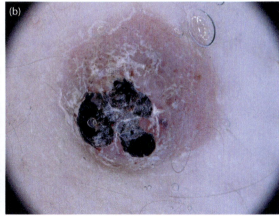

Figure 6.1 (a) Close-up of an amelanotic and ulcerated nodule arising on the extremity of an 11-year-old boy. (b) Dermatoscopy image of the lesion shows a nonspecific pattern, with polymorphic vessels, red and brown globules and a black crust.

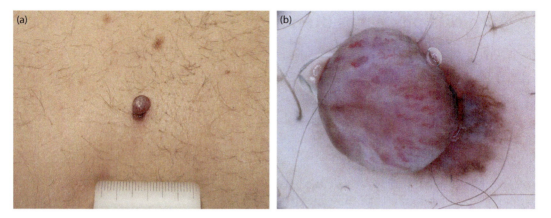

Figure 6.2 (a) Close-up of a red exophytic papule on the upper back of a 26-year-old man. (b) Dermatoscopy image of the lesion shows a pinkish to brownish background with polymorphous vessels on the exophytic portion, while the flat portion shows an irregular pigmented network with regression features.

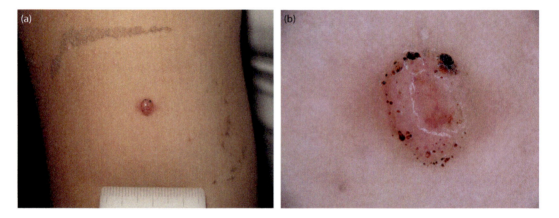

Figure 6.3 (a) Close-up of an amelanotic and partially ulcerated papule on the upper arm of an 8-year-old girl. (b) Dermatoscopy image of the lesion shows a pinkish background with irregular vessels and red globules.

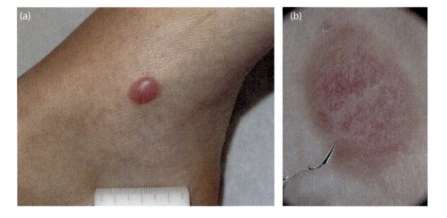

Figure 6.4 (a) Close-up image of a pinkish-red, well-defined plaque on the right ankle of a 19-year-old woman. (b) Dermatoscopy image of the lesion shows a nonspecific pattern, with polymorphic vessels and white lines visible over a pinkish background.

and "blue" tumors: the first one had a vascular pattern with dotted or polymorphous vessels, while the second appeared similar to blue nevi, with homogeneous blue pigmentation. Recently, Moscarella et al.[10] described clinical and dermoscopic features of a series of 55 ASTs. They observed that the majority of ASTs were nodular lesions; half of their cases were pigmented, and half were hypopigmented or nonpigmented. The most frequent dermoscopic pattern was the multicomponent pattern (Figures 6.1b and 6.2b), followed by a nonspecific pattern and a nonpigmented typical Spitzoid pattern (defined as a hypopigmented/amelanotic pattern with dotted vessels and/or reticular depigmentation) (Figures 6.3b and 6.4b).

REFERENCES

1. Kernen JA, Ackerman LV. Spindle cell nevi and epithelioid cell nevi (so-called juvenile melanomas) in children and adults: A clinicopathologic study of 27 cases. *Cancer*. 1960;**13**:612–25.
2. Smith KJ, Barrett TL, Skelton HG III et al. Spindle cell and epithelioid cell nevi with atypia and metastasis (malignant Spitz nevus). *Am J Surg Pathol*. 1989;**13**:931–9.
3. Barnhill RL, Flotte TJ, Fleischli M et al. Cutaneous melanoma and atypical Spitz tumors in children. *Cancer*. 1995;**76**:1833–45.
4. Barnhill RL, Argenyi ZB, From L et al. Atypical Spitz nevi/tumor: Lack of consensus for diagnosis, discrimination from melanoma, and prediction of outcome. *Hum Pathol*. 1999;**30**:513–20.
5. Mones JM, Ackerman AB. "Atypical" Spitz's nevus, "malignant" Spitz's nevus, and "metastasizing" Spitz's nevus: A critique in historical perspective of three concepts flawed fatally. *Am J Dermatopathol*. 2004;**26**:310–33.
6. Casso EM, Grin-Jorgensen CM, Grant-Kels JM. Spitz nevi. *J Am Acad Dermatol*. 1992;**27**:901–13.
7. Wiesner T, He J, Yelensky R et al. Kinase fusions are frequent in Spitz tumors and Spitzoid melanomas. *Nat Commun*. 2014;**5**:3116.
8. Ferrara G, Zalaudek I, Savarese I et al. Pediatric atypical Spitzoid neoplasms. A review with emphasis on "red" ("Spitz") tumors and "blue" ("Blitz") tumors. *Dermatology*. 2010;**220**:306–10.
9. Ludgate MW, Fullen DR, Lee J et al. The atypical Spitz tumor of uncertain biologic potential: A series of 67 patients from a single institution. *Cancer*. 2009;**115**:631.
10. Moscarella E, Lallas A, Kyrgidis A et al. Clinical and dermoscopic features of atypical Spitz tumors: A multicentre, retrospective, case-control study. *J Am Acad Dermatol*. 2015;**73**:777–84.
11. Elder DE, Xu X. The approach to the patient with a difficult melanocytic lesion. *Pathology*. 2004;**36**:428–34.
12. Zembowicz A, Scolyer RA. Nevus/melanocytoma/melanoma: An emerging paradigm for classification of melanocytic neoplasms? *Arch Pathol Lab Med*. 2011;**135**:300–6.
13. Massi D, De Giorgi V, Mandalà M. The complex management of atypical Spitz tumours. *Pathology*. 2016;**48**(2):132–41.
14. Lallas A, Kyrgidis A, Ferrara G. et al. Atypical Spitz tumours and sentinel lymph node biopsy: A systematic review. *Lancet Oncol*. 2014;**15**: e178–83.

7 Halo Spitz nevus

Caterina Bombonato

INTRODUCTION

The histologic spectrum of Spitz nevus is wide and many variants have been described, including pigmented spindle cell nevus of Reed, desmoplastic nevus, angiomatoid nevus, halo Spitz nevus and pagetoid nevus.[1-6] Few reports are present in literature, because in many cases only a "halo reaction" is visible (the term refers to nevi that demonstrate dense lymphocytic infiltrates histologically but lack clinical halos) without the presence of a clinical depigmentation (Figures 7.1 and 7.2).

Among the first cases reported was the case of Yasaka et al.[7] who described the halo phenomenon in a Spitz nevus in a 6-year-old girl. They observed that identical histopathological cellular mechanisms were involved in halo nevomelanocytic nevus and in halo Spitz nevus toward both the epidermal melanocytes and epithelioid nevus cells. These mechanisms lead to the destruction of melanocytes, resulting in depigmented halo and the destruction of nevus cells leading to regression of nevus. A few years later, Harvell and colleagues[8] reported 17 cases of Spitz's nevi with halo reaction and observed that, especially when this phenomenon occurred in a combined Spitz's nevus, it resembled melanomas. One must bear in mind that halo reactions may cause misdiagnosis of an otherwise benign nevus as melanoma because inflammatory cells sometimes obscure the architectural features of the underlying nevus and may induce cytologic atypia. For Spitz's nevus, where the distinction between malignancy and benignancy is already a challenge, halo reaction compounds the problem. Harvell et al. noted that architectural features of the underlying nevus, as well as the symmetry—or lack thereof—of the inflammatory cell infiltrate, help to distinguish it from malignant melanoma.

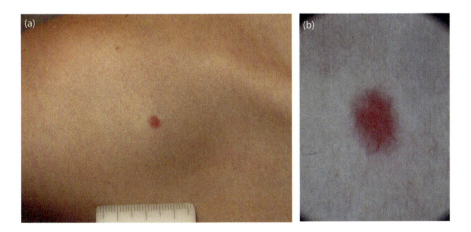

Figure 7.1 (a) Close-up image of a pinkish-red, well-defined papule on the right shoulder of a 14-year-old boy. (b) Dermatoscopy image of the lesion shows a pinkish-red background with few areas of thin, light-brown pigmented irregular network, dotted vessels and depigmentation all around.

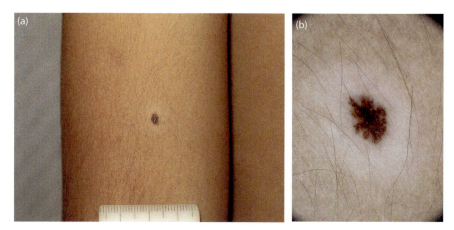

Figure 7.2 (a) Close-up image of brown lesion with a halo of depigmentation on the right arm of an 11-year-old boy. (b) Dermatoscopy image of the lesion shows an irregular pigmented network with globules surrounded by a border of depigmentation.

DERMOSCOPY

Clinical and dermoscopic features of unusual variants of Spitz nevi have been reported only rarely. Dermoscopy of halo Spitz nevus has not been reported until now.

REFERENCES

1. Busam KJ, Barnhill RL. Pagetoid Spitz nevus. Intraepidermal Spitz tumor with prominent pagetoid spread. *Am J Surg Pathol*. 1995;**19**:1061–7.
2. Reed RJ, Ichinose H, Clark WH Jr. et al. Common and uncommon melanocytic nevi and borderline melanomas. *Semin Oncol*. 1975;**2**:119–47.
3. Requena L, Sanchez Yus E. Pigmented spindle cell naevus. *Br J Dermatol*. 1990;**123**:757–63.
4. Requena C, Requena L, Kutzner H et al. Spitz nevus: A clinicopathological study of 349 cases. *Am J Dermatopathol*. 2009;**31**:107–16.
5. Barr RJ, Morales RV, Graham JH. Desmoplastic nevus: A distinct histologic variant of mixed spindle cell and epithelioid cell nevus. *Cancer*. 1980;**46**:557–64.
6. Tetzlaff MT, Xu X, Elder DE et al. Angiomatoid Spitz nevus: A clinicopathological study of six cases and a review of the literature. *J Cutan Pathol*. 2009;**36**:471–6.
7. Yasaka N, Furue M, Tamaki K. Histopathological evaluation of halo phenomenon in Spitz nevus. *Am J Dermatopathol*. 1995;**17**(5):484–6.
8. Harvell JD, Meehan SA, LeBoit PE. Spitz's nevi with halo reaction: A histopathologic study of 17 cases. *J Cutan Pathol*. 1997;**24**:611–9.

8 Desmoplastic nevus

Caterina Bombonato

INTRODUCTION

In 1980, Barr et al. described desmoplastic nevus as a distinct histologic entity, different from the Spitz nevus and not a manifestation of age-related changes as previously considered.[1] Desmoplastic (sclerotic) nevus is an infrequent, poorly characterized, benign melanocytic proliferation, with only a few case series published to date. Clinically, it usually presents as an asymptomatic, small (ranging between a few millimeters and 1 or 2 cm), flesh-colored, erythematous or slightly pigmented firm papule or nodule (Figures 8.1 through 8.3) that may be confused with other fibrous entities and

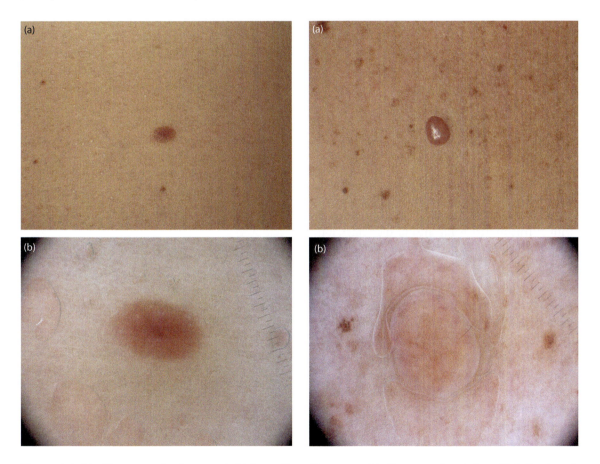

Figure 8.1 (a) Close-up of a brown-pinkish, well-defined macule. (b) Dermatoscopy image of the lesion shows a very light brown network in the center on a pinkish background.

Figure 8.2 (a) Close-up of a pink, well-defined nodule with a translucent surface. (b) Dermatoscopy image of the lesion shows a pinkish background with the presence of a small portion of brown network in the center.

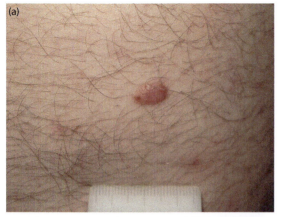

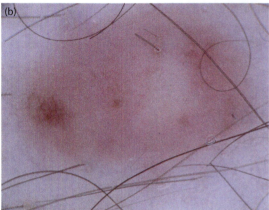

Figure 8.3 (a) Close-up of a pink papule with a brown portion at the periphery. (b) Dermatoscopy image of the lesion shows a pinkish background with a structureless white area in the center, a tiny brown network at the periphery and polymorphous vessels.

are removed because of a history of changes and because of their unusual dermatoscopic features. The main differential diagnosis is with desmoplastic melanoma, which is more frequently seen in older patients on sun-exposed areas.[5–6]

Some authors also report a rare variant of congenital nevus, called desmoplastic giant congenital melanocytic nevus (DGCN), presenting as a progressive induration and hypopigmentation of the lesion that occasionally causes hair loss and even a total or partial disappearance of the nevus.

DERMOSCOPY

Dermoscopically, only a few cases have been described, exhibiting a tiny, light brown network lying on a pinkish or brownish or erythematous background (Figures 8.1b through 8.3b). Scattered, small, brown globules were also visible in one of the cases reported. DGCN is usually symmetric in color and structure and without any melanoma-specific criteria.[7] The first dermoscopic description of DGCN was provided by Martin-Carrasco and colleagues.[8] They observed a typical reticular pattern in the perifollicular area, with a radial distribution from the follicular ostium on hypopigmented skin and described this pattern as a "sky full of stars."

atypical melanocytic proliferations including melanoma. It often occurs on the extremities of young adults (average age 30 years), with a female predominance. Histopathologically, it is characterized by spindle-shaped or epithelioid melanocytes, with readily appreciable pseudonucleoli embedded within a fibrotic stroma. It is included in the spectrum of dermal proliferations with a desmoplastic component composed by dermatofibroma, sclerotic blue nevus, desmoplastic nevus and desmoplastic melanoma. Their differentiation can sometimes represent a diagnostic dilemma for both clinicians and histopathologists.[2–4] In most of the cases, they

REFERENCES

1. Barr RJ, Morales RV, Graham JH. Desmoplastic nevus: A distinct histologic variant of mixed spindle cell and epithelioid cell nevus. *Cancer.* 1980;**46**:557–64.
2. Ferrara G, Brasiello M, Annese P et al. Desmoplastic nevus: Clinicopathologic keynotes. *Am J Dermatopathol.* 2009;**31**:718–22.
3. Mackie RM, Doherty VR. The desmoplastic melanocytic naevus: A distinct histological entity. *Histopathology.* 1992;**20**:207–11.
4. Meffert JJ, Peake MF, Wilde JL. "Dimpling" is not unique to dermatofibromas. *Dermatology.* 1997;**195**:384–6.
5. Sherrill AM, Crespo G, Prakash AV et al. Desmoplastic nevus: An entity distinct from Spitz nevus and blue nevus. *Am J Dermatopathol.* 2011;**33**(1):35–9.

6. Ruiz-Maldonado R, Orozco-Covarrubias L, Ridaura-Sanza C et al. Desmoplastic hairless hypopigmented nevus: A variant of giant congenital melanocytic naevus. *Br J Dermatol.* 2003;**148**(6):1253–7.
7. Larre Borges A, Zalaudek I, Longo C et al. Melanocytic nevi with special features: Clinical-dermoscopic and reflectance confocal microscopic-findings. *J Eur Acad Dermatol Venereol.* 2014;**28**(7):833–45.
8. Martin-Carrasco P, Bernabeu-Wittel J, Dominguez-Cruz J et al. "Sky full of stars" pattern: Dermoscopic findings in a desmoplastic giant congenital melanocytic nevus. *Pediatr Dermatol.* 2017;**34**(3):e142–3.

9 Pigmented epithelioid melanocytoma

Eugenia Veronica Di Brizzi, Gerardo Ferrara, Giuseppe Argenziano, and Elvira Moscarella

INTRODUCTION

Pigmented epithelioid melanocytoma (PEM) is an uncommon cutaneous melanocytic tumor described first by Zembowicz et al.[1] It shows overlapping features between an atypical epithelioid blue nevus and a low-grade animal-type melanoma. PEM can occur in patients with Carney complex (familial multiple neoplasia and lentiginous syndrome) but is more frequently seen as a sporadic lesion in patients without the complex.[1] PEMs show loss of expression of cyclic adenosine 3,5′ monophosphate (AMP)-dependent protein kinase A regulatory subunit 1α (R1α), a gene product associated with Carney complex. No loss of R1α was observed in blue nevi, melanoma or other melanocytic lesions. Loss of expression of R1α offers a useful diagnostic test that helps

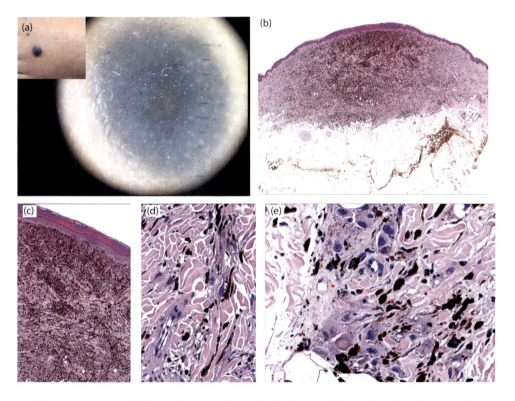

Figure 9.1 (a) Dermoscopy and clinical picture (insert) of a blue nodule on the foot dorsum of a 12-year-old male patient. (b–e) Homogeneous, structureless blue pigmentation is visible in dermoscopy with blue nevus-like features. (c) Histopathology: The neoplasm is horizontally oriented and heavily pigmented, with a thin grenz zone; (d, e) cytomorphologically, dendritic melanocytes are admixed with pleomorphic but mitotically inactive epithelioid cells.

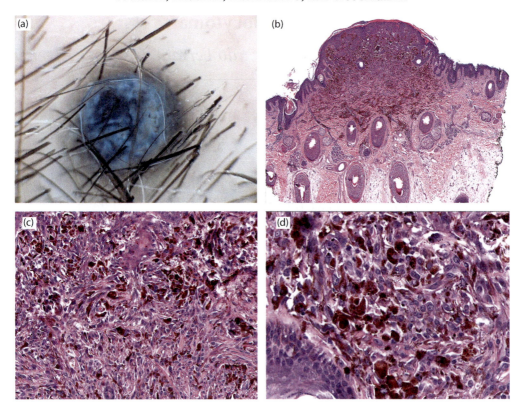

Figure 9.2 (a–d) Dermoscopy of a blue nodule on the scalp of a 32-year-old man. Blue color and white lines in the center of the lesion are visible. Histopathologically the neoplasm is nodular and heavily pigmented with pleomorphic atypical melanocytes.

to distinguish PEM from lesions that mimic it histologically.[2]

Clinically, PEM occurs more frequently as a slowly growing, dark papular or nodular lesion with blue-gray color, located on the face, trunk, extremities, conjunctiva and genital mucosa. Some lesions may be ulcerated or associated with epidermal hyperplasia and hyperkeratosis.

It shows a predilection for children and young patients, but ages range from infants to the elderly. It affects all races and both sexes. Involvement of the regional lymph nodes has been reported in up to 46% of cases, but usually with no further spread of the disease.[1,3–5] No histologic criteria are predictive of metastatic behavior.[1] Thus, the tumor could be a low-grade, lymphotropic variant of melanoma with frequent lymph node metastases but an indolent clinical course. Prognosis is good even in patients with metastatic deposits in sentinel lymph nodes.[1,3–5]

Histopathologically, it is characterized by dark pigment in deep derma with frequent involvement of subcutis and extension along the adnexal structures. It often presents hyperplasia of the epidermis above the tumor, and in some cases a grenz zone can be seen. PEMs are composed of several cell types. The first are spindled cells, some with pseudodendrites, small epithelioid cells with heavily pigmented cytoplasm and big epithelioid cells with big vesicles, eosinophilic macronuclei, light perinuclear cytoplasm and peripherally pigmented ring. Melanophages can be observed, constituting less than 10% of the cells in the tumor. Moreover, PEM shows prominent nuclear membrane and low mitotic activity.[3]

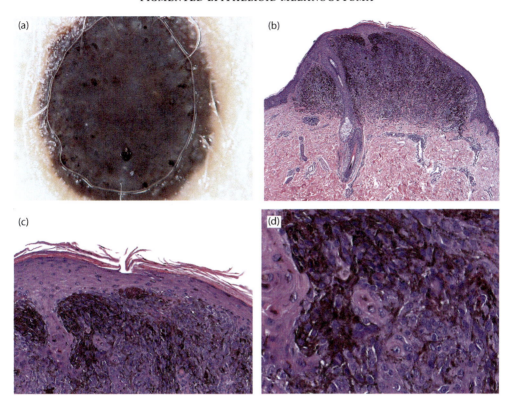

Figure 9.3 (a–d) Dermoscopy and histopathology of a heavily pigmented nodule arising on the back of an 11-year-old male. A dark brown and black pigmentation is visible in dermoscopy, with some structures resembling comedo-like openings.

The differentiating feature between PEM and blue nevi is the presence of abundant epithelioid cells in PEM, a feature not usually observed in blue nevi. Dermal sclerosis, common in blue nevus, is rarely seen in PEM.[3] The differential diagnosis between PEM and malignant blue nevus is the presence of high-grade cytologic atypia with high mitotic activity, atypical mitoses and tumor necrosis in malignant blue nevus.[3]

Other differential diagnoses include melanoma, Spitz nevus, atypical Spitz tumor, deep penetrating nevus and pigmented spindle cell nevus.

DERMOSCOPY

Dermoscopically, PEM shows homogeneous blue pigmentation and a variable combination of black, brown and white color. Sometimes the lesion presents a structureless blue pigmentation, or homogeneous blue and crystalline structures (Figures 9.1 through 9.3). In some lesions a bluish pigmentation in lymphatic vessels surrounding the tumor can be seen.[6]

Surgical excision with wide margins is always recommended. No further action is needed.

REFERENCES

1. Zembowicz A, Carney JA, Mihm MC. Pigmented epithelioid melanocytoma: A low-grade melanocytic tumor with metastatic potential indistinguishable from animal-type melanoma and epithelioid blue nevus. *Am J Surg Pathol.* 2004;**28**:31–40.
2. Zembrowicz A, Knoepp SM, Bei T et al. Loss of expression of protein kinase A regulatory subunit 1α in pigmented epithelioid melanocytoma but not in melanoma or other melanocytic lesions. *Am J Surg Pathol.* 2007;**31**(11):1764–75.

3. Ito K, Mihm MC. Pigmented epithelioid melanocytoma: Report of first Japanese cases previously diagnosed as cellular blue nevus. *J Cutan Pathol.* 2009;**36**(4):439–43.
4. Mandal RV, Murali R, Lundquist KF et al. Pigmented epithelioid melanocytoma: Favorable outcome after 5-year follow-up. *Am J Surg Pathol.* 2009;**33**:1778–82.
5. Lim C, Murali R, McCarthy SW et al. Pigmented epithelioid melanocytoma: A recently described melanocytic tumour of low malignant potential. *Pathology.* 2010;**42**:284–6.
6. Moscarella E, Ricci R, Argenziano G et al. Pigmented epithelioid melanocytoma: Clinical, dermoscopic and histopathological features. *Br J Dermatol.* 2016;**174**(5):1115–7.

10   Animal-type melanoma

Caterina Bombonato

INTRODUCTION

Animal-type melanoma (ATM) is so named because it is supposed to be similar to equine melanotic disease,[1] a long-lasting indolent form of melanoma with multiple lesions, particularly common in elderly, gray horses, which turn white after acquiring the disease. The similarity between this type of melanoma and that seen in humans was first noted by Darier, who introduced the term *melanosarcoma*.[2]

ATM is a controversial entity since some authors regard it as an entity in its own right, whereas others prefer to include it in the category of pigmented epithelioid melanocytoma (PEM) to reflect its apparent similarity to blue nevus as seen in Carney complex. It also shows considerable overlap with some examples of malignant blue nevus.[3,4]

It is associated with a wide age range, although most patients are in the third or fourth decades. Congenital or very early cases are on record as well.[5,6] Caucasians are most often affected, and the genders are affected equally. The head and neck represent the most common sites.[7]

It appears as heavily pigmented, dark brown, blue or black dome-shaped or verrucous nodules, 1 cm or more in diameter (Figures 10.1 and 10.2) and often of long duration since they appear many years before the diagnosis, even if there are fast-growing cases. Satellite lesions are relatively common (Figure 10.1). Histopathologically, the lesion consists of a large, homogeneously, pigmented black mass of atypical melanocytes and melanophages located in the dermis and often reaches and extends into the subcutis. It is asymmetric and poorly demarcated. There is a tendency to infiltrate and destroy the follicular structures. It is composed of epithelioid, spindled and dendritic or "pseudodendritic" cells with vesicular and hyperchromatic nuclei. Mitotic figures are also present.[7]

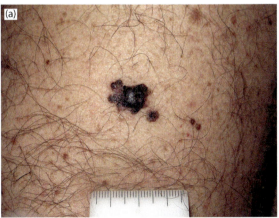 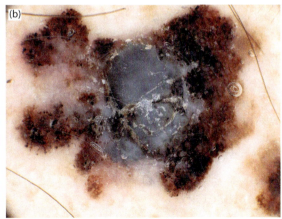

Figure 10.1 (a) Close-up of brown-black nodule on the arm of a 46-year-old man. (b) Dermatoscopy image of the lesion shows a homogeneous blue-black pattern, irregular whitish/pinkish structureless area at the periphery, and an irregular pigment network with clods, globules and blotches.

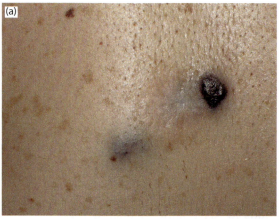
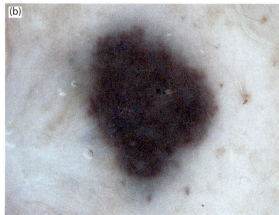
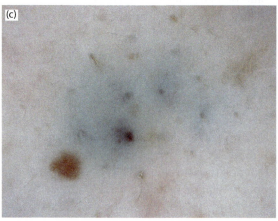

Figure 10.2 (a) Close-up of a blue-black nodule on the upper back of a 44-year-old woman at the periphery of a scar area of a previous surgery. (b) Dermatoscopy image of the lesion shows a homogeneous blue-black network on a brown background on one side of the scar. A blue-white veil is also present. (c) Dermatoscopy image of the other side of the scar shows a bluish subcutaneous pigmentation with a blue-brown globule.

Nodal spread is common since the sentinel lymph node is positive in 30%–47% of cases and additional lymph nodes are occasionally found on completion of lymphadenectomy, but distant metastases are rare. Also, the metastases have a slow growth rate, and the mortality appears to be extremely low.[3,7]

ATM should be distinguished from heavily pigmented conventional melanoma, heavily pigmented metastatic melanoma, pigmented epithelioid melanocytoma, tumoral (or nodular) melanosis and melanoma with features of blue nevus.[8–10]

DERMOSCOPY

Dermoscopically, only three cases have been described up to now by Avilés-Izquiedo and colleagues.[11] In their series all lesions showed a homogeneous blue pattern, irregular whitish structures and a polymorphous vascular pattern generally composed of large, irregular vessels (Figures 10.1b and 10.2b, c). These dermoscopic features, however, are not specific to ATM and therefore cannot be used to differentiate between this type of melanoma and any other dermal melanocytic proliferations.[11]

REFERENCES

1. Dick W. Melanosis in men and horses (letter). *Lancet*. 1832;192.
2. Darier J. Le melanoma malin mesenchymateaux ou melanosarcome. *Bull Assoc Fr Cancer*. 1925;**14**:221–49.
3. Zembowicz A, Carney JA, Mihm MC. Pigmented epithelioid melanocytoma: A low-grade melanocytic tumor with metastatic potential indistinguishable from animal-type melanoma and epithelioid blue nevus. *Am J Surg Pathol*. 2004;**28**:31–40.

4. Mandal RV, Murali R, Lundquist KFA et al. Pigmented epithelioid melanocytoma: Favorable outcome after 5-year follow-up. *Am J Surg Pathol.* 2009;**33**:1778–82.
5. Richardson SK, Tannous ZS, Mihm MC. Congenital and infantile melanoma: Review of the literature and report of an uncommon variant, pigment-synthesizing melanoma. *J Am Acad Dermatol.* 2002;**47**:77–90.
6. Yun SJ, Han DK, Lee MC et al. Congenital pigment synthesizing melanoma of the scalp. *J Am Acad Dermatol.* 2010;**62**(2):324–9.
7. Antony FC, Sanclemente G, Shaikh H et al. Pigment synthesizing melanoma (so-called animal type melanoma): A clinicopathological study of 14 of a poorly known distinctive variant of melanoma. *Histopathology.* 2006;**48**(6):754–62.
8. Granter SR, McKee PH, Calonje E et al. Melanoma associated with blue nevus and melanoma mimicking a cellular blue nevus: A clinicopathologic study of 10 cases on the spectrum of so-called "malignant blue nevus." *Am J Surg Pathol.* 2001;**25**:316–23.
9. Seab JA Jr, Graham JH, Helwig EB. Deep penetrating nevus. *Am J Surg Pathol.* 1989;**13**:39–44.
10. Robson A, Morley-Quante M, Hempel H et al. Deep penetrating naevus: Clinicopathological study of 31 cases with further delineation of histological features allowing distinction from other pigmented benign melanocytic lesions and melanoma. *Histopathology.* 2003;**43**:529–37.
11. Avilés-Izquierdo JA, Leis-Dosil VM, Lázaro-Ochaita P. Animal-type melanoma: Clinical and dermoscopic features of 3 cases. *Actas Dermosifiliogr.* 2014;**105**(2):186–90.

11 Nevoid melanoma

Caterina Bombonato

INTRODUCTION

Nevoid melanoma (NeM) is an uncommon subtype of malignant melanoma included among the less frequent variants and it can be very difficult to differentiate clinically and histologically from nevi.[1-6] Clinically, it presents as a variously pigmented papillomatous (Figure 11.1a) or dome-shaped papule or nodule (Figures 11.2a and 11.3a) that is often greater than 1 cm in diameter and is located on the trunk and on the limbs. The verrucous appearance of the nevoid melanoma can deceptively evoke a benign diagnosis of dermal or compound nevus, seborrheic keratosis or papilloma. There is a male predominance and mean age of patients is 51–57 years.[5-8] Histologically, subtle clues that enable NeM to be differentiated from benign melanocytic lesions are the presence of multiple dermal mitoses, often deep and atypical, nucleolar prominence, subtle pleomorphism, slight asymmetry and impaired circumscription.[5,8] Furthermore, when the tumor cells are small, NeM mimics ordinary compound nevus or dermal nevi; when cells are large, NeM mimics Spitz nevi.[5]

DERMOSCOPY

The paper by Longo et al. gives new insights into the dermoscopic features of NeM.[9] The global dermoscopic pattern can be classified into one of three distinct types: nevus-like tumors, amelanotic tumors and tumors with a multicomponent pattern.

Into the first group they classified lesions showing a papillomatous or mammilated surface with a cobblestone dermoscopic pattern that revealed irregular dots/globules, irregular pigmentation, an atypical vascular

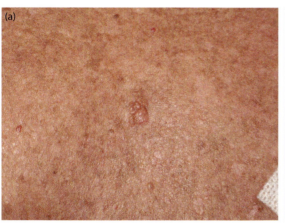 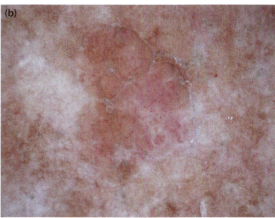

Figure 11.1 (a) Close-up of a skin-colored papillomatous plaque. (b) Dermatoscopy image of the lesion shows a structureless pinkish area with an irregular distribution of polymorphous vessels. A rim of brown pigmentation is present in the upper part.

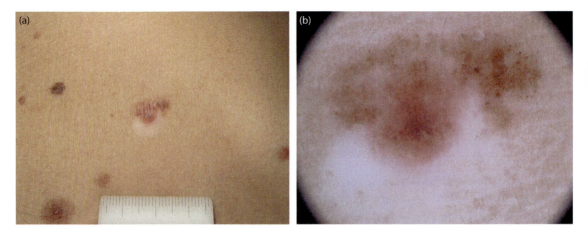

Figure 11.2 (a) Close-up of a multicolored plaque that appears to be composed of distinct parts. (b) Dermatoscopy image of the lesion shows dots and globules and structureless white areas. Multiple colors and polymorphous vessels are seen.

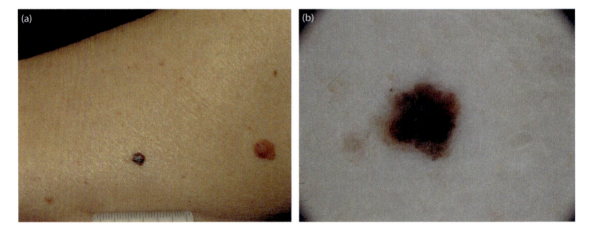

Figure 11.3 (a) Close-up of a dark brown nodule on the right arm. (b) Dermatoscopy image of the lesion shows a multicomponent pattern: A blue veil with scar-like areas, brown globules, black blotches.

pattern with polymorphic vessels and multiple milia-like cysts (Figures 11.1b and 11.2b) (features often associated with benign lesion). In the second group, they included lesions lacking significant pigmentation with a predominantly atypical vascular pattern consisting of linear irregular, dotted and/or glomerular vessels. In the third group, they included lesions revealing the classical melanoma-specific criteria, such as blue-white veil, irregular pigmentation and an atypical network (Figure 11.3b).

REFERENCES

1. Levene A. On the histological diagnosis and prognosis of malignant melanoma. *J Clin Pathol.* 1980;**33**:101–24.
2. Schmoeckel C, Castro CE, Braun-Falco O. Nevoid malignant melanoma. *Arch Dermatol Res.* 1985;**277**:362–9.
3. Suster S, Ronnen M, Bubis JJ. Verrucous pseudonevoid melanoma. *J Surg Oncol.* 1987;**36**:134–7.
4. Wong T, Suster S, Duncan LM, Mihm MC. Nevoid melanoma: A clinicopathological study of seven cases of malignant melanoma mimicking

spindle and epithelioid cell nevus and verrucous dermal nevus. *Hum Pathol.* 1995;**26**:171–9.

5. McNutt NS, Urmacher C, Hakimian J et al. Nevoid malignant melanoma: Morphologic patterns and immunohistochemical reactivity. *J Cutan Pathol.* 1995;**22**:502–17.

6. Zembowicz A, McCusker M, Chiarelli C et al. Morphological analysis of nevoid melanoma: A study of 20 cases with a review of the literature. *Am J Dermatopathol.* 2001;**23**:167–75.

7. McNutt NS. "Triggered trap": Nevoid malignant melanoma. *Semin Diagn Pathol.* 1998;**15**:203–9.

8. Kossard S, Wilkinson B. Small cell (naevoid) melanoma: A clinicopathologic study of 131 cases. *Australas J Dermatol.* 1997;**38**:54–8.

9. Longo C, Piana S, Marghoob A et al. Morphological features of naevoid melanoma: Results of a multicentre study of the International Dermoscopy Society. *Br J Dermatol.* 2015;**172**(4):961–7.

12 Balloon cell melanoma

Caterina Bombonato

INTRODUCTION

Balloon cell malignant melanoma (BCMM) has been described as the rarest histologic type of primary cutaneous melanoma and is composed of large, polyhedral, foamy cells with abundant cytoplasmic vacuoles.[1,2] The first case was reported in 1970 by Gardner and Vazquez.[3] The clinical presentation is variable: nodular, ulcerated, pedunculated, polypoid, papillomatous and often nonpigmented (Figures 12.1 and 12.2).

The clinical differential diagnosis includes halo nevus, Spitz nevus, dermatofibroma, fibromatous lesions, malignant melanoma, basal cell carcinoma, squamous cell carcinoma and cutaneous adnexal tumors.

Histologically, it can present with four cell types: balloon melanoma cells (BMCs), spindle-shaped or epithelioid melanoma cells, transitional cells and conventional nevi cells.[4] The BCMM must be composed of more than 50% of foamy cells.[2] In the primary lesions, BMCs are usually sparse or absent; however, when it metastasizes, the metastases are often composed entirely of balloon cells with no residual spindle-shaped or epithelioid component. Immunohistochemistry is helpful in the diagnosis, in conjunction with clinical history and other diagnostic modalities. The prognosis does not depend on the degree of balloon cells change, tumor size, nuclear atypia or mitotic activity, but instead follows the prognosis patterns of conventional malignant melanoma correlating with tumor thickness. The mortality rate is reported to be higher than other subtypes of melanoma, probably due to the fact that BCMM tends to be thick at the time of presentation.

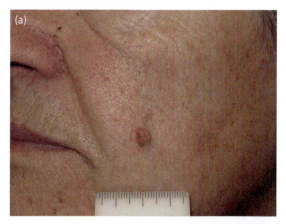
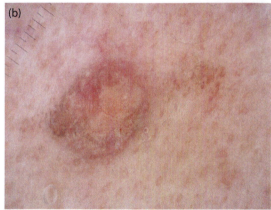

Figure 12.1 Close-up of an erythematous, pinkish nodule on the left cheek of a 76-year-old woman. There are foci of eccentric pigmentation and scales at the periphery. (b) Dermatoscopy image of the lesion shows a structureless white-yellow area with a rim of structureless brown containing focal reticular lines, a focal pattern of dot vessels in the center and polymorphous vessels in the upper periphery.

DERMOSCOPY

Inskip and colleagues[5] were the first to describe the dermoscopic pattern of a BCMM, observed in a 68-year-old man. Dermoscopically, the

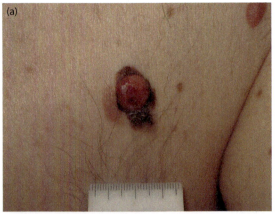

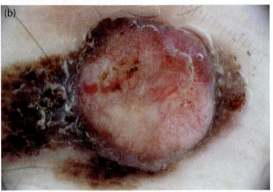

Figure 12.2 (a) Close-up of an erythematous nodule surrounded by brown and light brown pigmentation on the upper back of a 68-year-old man. (b) Dermatoscopy image of the lesion shows a structureless, white central area with polymorphous vessels all over the nodular part. Shown at the periphery is a brown irregular pigmentation with globules, clods and blotches.

lesion was a nonpigmented, structureless yellow with three terminal hairs emanating from it and an erythematous central part corresponding to the ulceration caused by the prior trauma reported by the patient. Vessels observed were very sparse. None of the specific clues of melanoma were observed (Figure 12.1b).

Maher et al.[6] reported the second dermoscopic description of a BCMM. They observed dermatoscopic asymmetry of structures and color (white and brown), polymorphous vessels (linear curved vessels and dots vessels) and chrysalis structures (Figure 12.2b). To date, cases reported were amelanotic.

Han and colleagues[1] described a case report of BCMM presenting as a black nodule without describing the dermoscopic pattern, while Inskip and colleagues[7] described the first published dermatoscopic pigmented case of BCMM. They observed a structureless pattern with two colors, blue-gray centrally and brown peripherally, almost symmetrically combined as well as with reticular lines in association with a polymorphous vessels pattern with linear, dot and serpentine vessels.

REFERENCES

1. Han JS, Won CH, Chang SE et al. Primary cutaneous balloon cell melanoma: A very rare variant. *Int J Dermatol.* 2014;**53**:e535–6.
2. Kao GF, Helwig EB, Graham JH. Balloon cell malignant melanoma of the skin. A clinicopathologic study of 34 cases with histochemical, immunohistochemical, and ultrastructural observations. *Cancer.* 1992;**69**:2942–52.
3. Gardner WA Jr, Vazquez MD. Balloon cell melanoma. *Arch Pathol.* 1970;**89**:470–2.
4. Lee L, Zhou F, Simms A et al. Metastatic balloon cell malignant melanoma: A case report and literature review. *Int J Clin Exp Pathol.* 2011;**4**(3):315–21.
5. Inskip M, Magee J, Barksdale S et al. Balloon cell melanoma in primary care practice: A case report. *Dermatol Pract Concept.* 2013;**3**(3):6.
6. Maher J, Cameron A, Wallace S et al. Balloon cell melanoma: A case report with polarized and nonpolarized dermatoscopy and dermatopathology. *Dermatol Pract Concept.* 2014;**4**(1):69–73.
7. Inskip M, James N, Magee J et al. Pigmented primary cutaneous balloon cell melanoma demonstrating balloon cells in the dermoepidermal junction: A brief case report with dermatoscopy and histopathology. *Int J Dermatol.* 2016;**55**(2):e110–2.

13   Desmoplastic melanoma

Caterina Bombonato

INTRODUCTION

Desmoplastic melanoma (DM) is an uncommon variant of spindle cell melanoma, accounting for less than 4% of all melanomas.[1] The overall incidence rate of DM is 2.0 per million, with a peak of 15.2 per million for persons 80 years old or older. The male-to-female ratio for DM is approximately 2:1, and the mean age at diagnosis is 66 years.[2]

Chronic ultraviolet (UV) exposure has been linked to DM, and this may account for the distribution pattern, with approximately half of DM found on the head and neck, extremities and trunk.

The diagnosis of DM is challenging since its clinical presentation is often nonspecific.

Clinically, DM often presents as amelanotic nodules or plaques, or as ill-defined scar-like lesions (Figures 13.1 and 13.2).

The differential diagnosis is broad and includes scar, dermatofibroma, neurofibroma or malignant lesions, such as basal cell carcinoma, squamous cell carcinoma and amelanotic melanoma.[3]

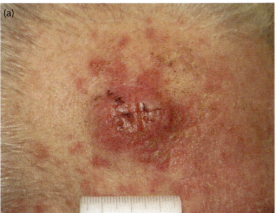
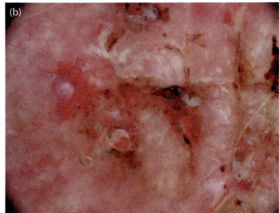
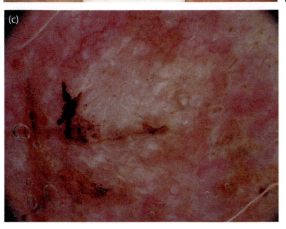

Figure 13.1 (a) Close-up of a pinkish nodule on the forehead that previously underwent a biopsy. (b, c) Dermatoscopy images of the lesion show white and pink colors without any specific pattern.

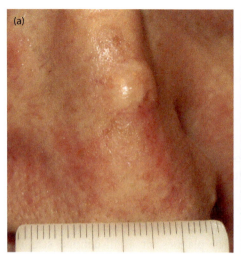 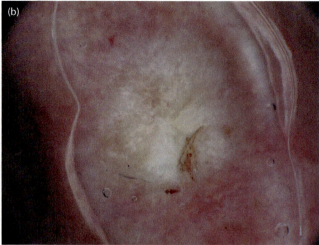

Figure 13.2 (a) Close-up of a whitish, well-defined nodule on the nose. (b) Dermatoscopy image of the lesion shows the predominance of white scar-like color with a little erosion in the lower part.

DM can arise *de novo* or in association with other melanoma subtypes, most often of the lentigo maligna type. Given its association with lentigo maligna melanoma (LMM), it is advisable to palpate the skin suspected of LMM to detect any firm subcutaneous nodule that may point to DM.[4]

The term DM initially referred to the association of invasive tumor cells with abundant stromal collagen but has been further classified into two histopathologic subtypes—pure DM (pDM) and mixed DM (mDM)—based on the degree of desmoplasia present in the tumor.[5] Patients with pDM less frequently have node involvement and tend to have a less aggressive clinical course than patients with mDM.

It differs from other subtypes of melanoma by having a higher tendency for persistent local growth and less frequent nodal metastasis. The 5-year overall survival (OS) for DM ranges between 67% and 89%.[6] Advancing age, male gender and head and neck location are associated with an increased risk of DM-specific death. Controversy persists regarding the prognosis of DM compared with nondesmoplastic melanomas.

The first line of treatment for any primary cutaneous melanoma is surgical management, but since DM frequently affects the head and neck region, cosmetic and anatomic restraints may prevent excision with adequate margins. In addition, higher recurrence rates have been attributed to nerve involvement because surgical margins may fail to detect focal persistent tumor deposits around nerve trunks. The predilection for local recurrence and neurotropism supports the current guidelines that wider margins of at least 2 cm are preferred for DM.[4]

Sentinel lymph node biopsy may be unnecessary for patients with pDM; however, it should be considered in patients with mDM, especially in those manifesting high-risk DM tumor characteristics such as deep infiltration, neurotropism, ulceration and/or higher mitotic rate.

Following surgery, adjuvant radiotherapy appears beneficial in patients with locally recurrent DM, residual gross tumors, DM with perineural involvement or DM excised with narrow margins.

DERMOSCOPY

The diagnosis of DM is challenging because its clinical presentation is often aspecific. For these reasons, there is limited information about its dermoscopic characteristics (Figures 13.1b, c and 13.2b).

Debarbieux and colleagues examined the dermoscopic presentation of six patients with DM.[7] They observed that for hypopigmented or amelanotic lesions, the presence of white, scar-like structureless areas and abnormal vascular patterns, such as linear-irregular vessels (also known as serpentine vessels) and milky-red areas were the only potential visual clues.

Jaimes and colleagues[8] analyzed 37 cases of DM and observed that 43% of the lesions revealed melanocytic structures, including atypical globules, atypical pigment network, polygonal lines and an asymmetric annular granular pattern. All of the lesions revealed at least one melanoma-specific structure, particularly atypical vascular structures and regression structures such as peppering.

REFERENCES

1. Quinn MJ, Crotty KA, Thompson JF et al. Desmoplastic and desmoplastic neurotropic melanoma: Experience with 280 patients. *Cancer.* 1998;**83**:1128–35.
2. Feng Z, Wu X, Chen V et al. Incidence and survival of desmoplastic melanoma in the United States, 1992–2007. *J Cutan Pathol.* 2011;**38**:616–24.
3. Busam KJ. Desmoplastic melanoma. *Clin Lab Med.* 2011;**31**:321–30.
4. Chen LL, Jaimes N, Barker CA et al. Desmoplastic melanoma: A review. *J Am Acad Dermatol.* 2013;**68**(5):825–33.
5. Busam KJ, Mujumdar U, Hummer AJ et al. Cutaneous desmoplastic melanoma: Reappraisal of morphologic heterogeneity and prognostic factors. *Am J Surg Pathol.* 2004;**28**:1518–25.
6. Wasif N, Gray RJ, Pockaj BA. Desmoplastic melanoma—The step-child in the melanoma family? *J Surg Oncol.* 2011;**103**:158–62.
7. Debarbieux S, Ronger-Salve S, Dalle S et al. Dermoscopy of desmoplastic melanoma: Report of six cases. *Br J Dermatol.* 2008;**159**:360–3.
8. Jaimes N, Chen L, Dusza WA et al. Clinical and dermoscopic characteristics of desmoplastic melanomas. *JAMA Dermatol.* 2013;**149**(4):413–21.

14 Special site melanoma (mucosal, acral)

Caterina Bombonato

INTRODUCTION

Primary cutaneous melanoma arising in the mucosal areas is a rare clinical entity that represents 1%–8% of all melanomas. There is higher prevalence in Asians than in Caucasians, and it has an extremely poor prognosis. Early detection and a wide excision provide the best likelihood of a favorable outcome.

Sinonasal mucosal melanoma presents with unilateral nasal obstruction, epistaxis, or a combination of the two. Discharge, epiphora, facial pain and swelling are more common in advanced cases.

Oral melanomas usually present on the hard palate, maxillary gingiva and lips. Most patients are in the seventh decade. The clinical presentation of tumors is variable, from macular to ulcerated and nodular painless mass, often bleeding. The colors vary from black to gray to purple to red to white, and they can be variably arranged. Pigmented lesions from 1 to 10 mm or larger can be found, and reports of previously existing pigmented lesions are common. Amelanotic melanoma cases are also reported, and in these cases a misdiagnosis is frequent. The differential diagnosis for intraoral melanotic lesions includes mucosal melanoma, amalgam tattoo, melanotic macule, oral mucosal nevi and melanoacanthoma.

Mucosal melanomas of the genital tract can occur on the glans, vagina and vulva (on the labia minora or clitoris). Early mucosal melanoma of the genital tract clinically presents as brown-black macules with shades of gray (Figure 14.1). The diameter is larger than 1 cm, and multifocal growth is possible. Advanced mucosal melanoma presents as black or brown nodules combined frequently with the macular

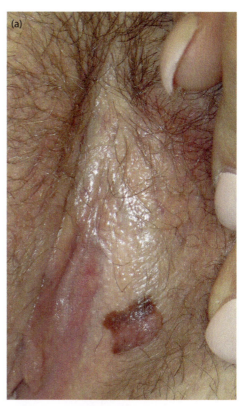

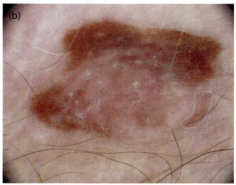

Figure 14.1 (a) Close-up of a vulvar melanoma in a young woman. (b) Dermatoscopy image of the lesion shows an irregular pigment network with prevalence of brown and pink colors and white areas.

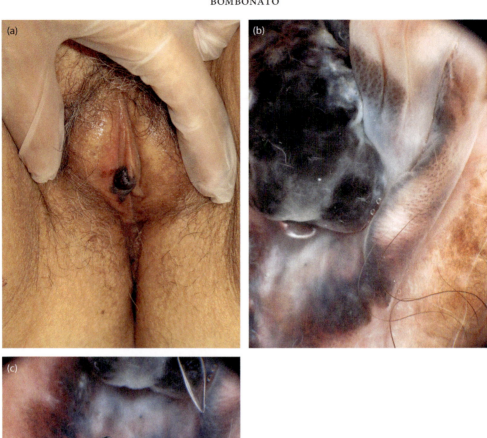
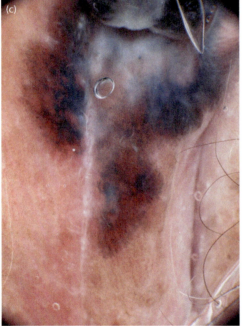

Figure 14.2 (a) Close-up of vulvar melanoma in a 65-year-old woman. (b, c) Dermatoscopy image of the lesion shows a black nodule with blue and white colors (b); at the periphery, the flat pigmentation is irregular; black, blue and white colors are present (c).

part at the basis of a tumor (Figure 14.2). In cases of amelanotic melanoma, red is the dominant color. Early stages of mucosal melanoma can be in differential diagnosis with benign melanotic macules.

Acral melanoma (AM) is a rare subtype of malignant melanoma arising on acral skin, primarily on the soles of the feet, palms of the hands and the nail beds. The prognosis is extremely poor because of the more advanced stage of presentation at diagnosis. It clinically presents as blue-black macules (Figure 14.3) or a nodule with irregular borders on acral skin. Amelanotic lesions appear as pinkish-red

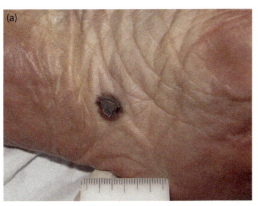 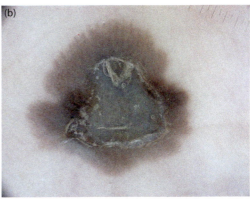

Figure 14.3 (a) Close-up of an acral melanoma in a 91-year-old woman. (b) Dermatoscopy image of the lesion shows a homogenous brown pattern with black and gray in the center of the lesion.

macules or nodules. The differential diagnosis includes acral nevus, pyoderma gangrenosum, pyogenic granuloma, verrucous carcinoma and peripheral neuropathy–induced foot ulcers. The subungual lesions clinically appear as melanonychia striata in the nail plate, larger than two-thirds of the nail plate, which continue as a dark pigmentation onto the proximal or lateral nail fold (Hutchinson's sign) (Figure 14.4).

DERMOSCOPY

There are limited studies on the dermoscopic features of mucosal melanoma, and they are focused mostly on vulvar melanoma (VM), but given the low incidence of this entity, most of the information is derived from small retrospective case series and single-case reports.

Blum et al. observed 11 cases of VM characterized by the presence of blue, gray or white colors with or without structureless areas.[1] De Giorgi et al. observed a case of VM with a blue-gray area and whitish veil.[2] Lin and colleagues described two cases of VM and observed a multicomponent pattern with multiple colors and blue-white veil.[3] In a case report of VM, Rogers et al. observed a brown-black pigmentation with structureless areas and central blue and pink colors.[4] Resende et al. presented two cases of VM and reviewed the literature: they concluded that dermoscopic patterns of VM do not differ from melanomas at other body sites,[5] especially if there is the presence of blue and black or blue with colors or polymorphic vessels (Figures 14.1b and 14.2b, c).

Even if the parallel ridge pattern is considered the hallmark of acral melanoma,[6] for AM appearing on weight-bearing areas of the body such as the soles, dermoscopy reveals an irregular fibrillar pattern showing structureless pigmentation instead of a parallel ridge pattern, which is believed to be due to shift in the horny layer.[7] Studies confirm that the most prevalent patterns found in volar AM are the parallel ridge pattern and irregular diffuse pigmentation, while amelanotic AM shows remnants of pigmentation and a polymorphic vascular pattern.[8] However, as highlighted by a recent study, all classic melanoma criteria can be present on an acral site (Figure 14.3b).[9]

In a recent study, Benati et al.[10] described dermoscopic features of nail melanoma. They observed that nail melanoma involved more than two-thirds of the nail plate, gray and black colors were the most frequent, there was irregularity of the line that composed the pigmented band and Hutchinson's and micro-Hutchinson's signs were often present (Figure 14.4b, c). Also, nail dystrophy was found frequently. A new criterion, granular pigmentation, was also present.

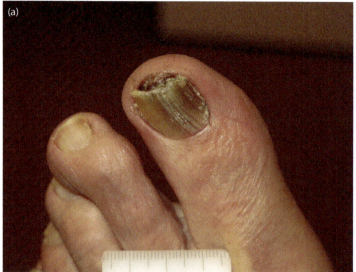
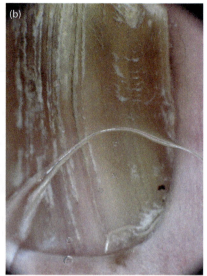
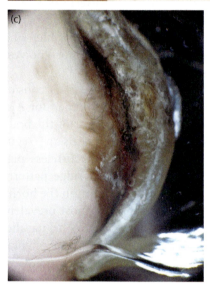

Figure 14.4 (a) Close-up of a nail melanoma in a man. (b, c) Dermatoscopy image of the lesion shows an irregular brown pigmentation larger than two-thirds of the nail surface (b) and an irregular brown pigmentation of the nail plate (c).

REFERENCES

1. Blum A, Simionescu O, Argenziano G et al. Dermoscopy of pigmented lesions of the mucosa and the mucocutaneous junction: Results of a multicenter study by the International Dermoscopy Society (IDS). *Arch Dermatol.* 2011;**147**(10):1181–7.
2. de Giorgi V, Massi D, Salvini C et al. Thin melanoma of the vulva: A clinical, dermoscopic-pathologic case study. *Arch Dermatol.* 2005;**141**(8):1046–7.
3. Lin J, Koga H, Takata M et al. Dermoscopy of pigmented lesions on mucocutaneous junction and mucous membrane. *Br J Dermatol.* 2009;**161**(6):1255–61.
4. Rogers T, Pulitzer M, Marino ML et al. Early diagnosis of genital mucosal melanoma: How good are our dermoscopic criteria? *Dermatol Pract Concept.* 2016;**6**(4):10–1.
5. Resende FS, Conforti C, Giuffrida R et al. Raised vulvar lesions: Be aware! *Dermatol Pract Concept.* 2018;**8**(2):16.
6. Saida T, Koga H, Uhara H. Key points in dermoscopic differentiation between early acral melanoma and acral nevus. *J Dermatol.* 2011;**38**:25–34.

7. Watanabe S, Sawada M, Ishizaki S et al. Comparison of dermatoscopic images of acral lentiginous melanoma and acral melanocytic nevus occurring on body weight-bearing areas. *Dermatol Pract Concept*. 2014;**4**:47–50.
8. Phan A, Dalle S, Touzet S et al. Dermoscopic features of acral lentiginous melanoma in a large series of 110 cases in a white population. *Br J Dermatol*. 2010;**162**:765–71.
9. Lallas A, Kyrgidis A, Koga H et al. The BRAAF checklist: A new dermoscopic algorithm for diagnosing acral melanoma. *Br J Dermatol*. 2015;**173**:1041–9.
10. Benati E, Ribero S, Longo C et al. Clinical and dermoscopic clues to differentiate pigmented nail bands: An International Dermoscopy Society study. *JEADV*. 2017;**31**:732–6.

SECTION III

Tumors of Cutaneous Appendages

15 Trichoadenoma

Riccardo Pampena

INTRODUCTION

Trichoadenoma is a rare benign tumor of the hair follicle, which was first described in 1958 by Nikolowski as "organoid follicular hamartoma."[1] It commonly presents as a solitary flesh-colored papule, usually not exceeding 1.5 cm in diameter and generally involving adults, with no sex predilection.[2] More than half of cases have been described on the face and almost one-quarter on the buttocks; however, other body regions, including the genital area, may also be affected.[3] On clinical ground, trichoadenoma is generally indistinguishable from other more common skin lesions, in particular, basal cell carcinoma (BCC).[4] Histologically, trichoadenoma corresponds to a well-circumscribed, dermal nodule, with no continuity with the overlying epidermis. The tumor typically consists of multiple infundibulocystic structures lined with stratified squamous epithelium, showing epidermoid keratinization toward the central cavity. A poorly developed fibrous stroma surrounds these structures, and solid cords of basaloid or infundibular cells projecting from

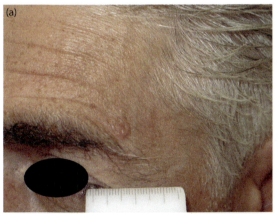
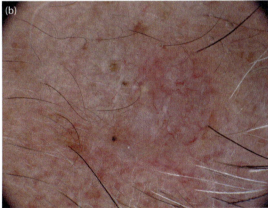
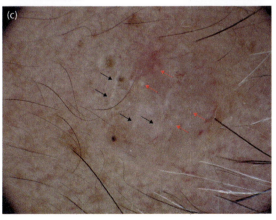

Figure 15.1 (a) Clinical picture revealing a 5-mm flesh-colored papule on the left eyebrow of a 45-year-old man. (b, c) Dermoscopic pictures with polarized light, without (b) and with (c) compression. In-focus linear vessels may be seen when compression was not applied; in addition, ovoidal blue-gray areas were visible at the periphery of the tumor. When compression was not applied, white structures were more visible, in particular, shiny white lines (black arrows) and small whitish circles (red arrows).

the cystic wall within the stroma are commonly found. Calcifications and hair shaft are typically absent.[5] The histopathologic appearance resembles multiple cross sections of the infundibular portion of hair follicles.

DERMOSCOPY

To the best of our knowledge, no reports in the literature have described the dermoscopic aspects of trichoadenoma. We report a case of histologically confirmed trichoadenoma in a 45-year-old man who came to our attention for a long-standing, 5-mm flesh-colored papule on the external edge of his left eyebrow (Figure 15.1a). The lesion was firm and painless and was excised with the suspicion of BCC. On dermoscopic examination, the tumor was mainly characterized by BCC-specific criteria; indeed, both in-focus linear vessels and shiny white lines could be identified, also involving the central area. In addition, an ovoidal blue-gray area was also visible at the periphery of the tumor. However, another dermoscopic feature could also be found, which is not typically seen in BCC, consisting of small whitish circles spread throughout the lesion. The histopathological correlate of this finding could be represented by infundibulocystic structures (Figure 15.1b, c).

REFERENCES

1. Nikolowski W. Trichoadenom (organoides Follikel-Hamartom). *Arch Klin Exp Dermatol.* 1958;**207**:34–45.
2. Lee JH, Kim YY, Yoon SY, Lee JD, Cho SH. Unusual presentation of trichoadenoma in an infant. *Acta Derm Venereol.* 2008;**88**:291–2.
3. Krishna Swaroop DS, Ramakrishna BA, Bai SJ, Shanthi V. Trichoadenoma of Nikolowski. *Indian J Pathol Microbiol.* 2008;**51**:277–9.
4. Tellechea O, Cardoso JC, Reis JP, Ramos L, Gameiro AR, Coutinho I, Baptista AP. Benign follicular tumors. *An Bras Dermatol.* 2015;**90**(6):780–96;quiz 797–8.
5. Shimanovich I, Krahl D, Rose C. Trichoadenoma of Nikolowski is a distinct neoplasm within the spectrum of follicular tumors. *J Am Acad Dermatol.* 2010;**62**:277–83.

16 Trichoepithelioma

Riccardo Pampena

INTRODUCTION

Trichoepithelioma is an uncommon benign tumor deriving from the hair germ, which may be mainly seen in adults as a solitary skin-colored papule, up to 0.5 cm in diameter, and mainly located on the nose, upper lip and cheeks.[1] Besides the less uncommon solitary form, two other variants have been described: multiple and desmoplastic. The latter is now considered as a distinct clinicopathologic entity with specific histopathologic features and is discussed separately in Chapter 17; on the contrary, multiple trichoepitheliomas are identical to the solitary form on histopathologic examination but typically involve younger individuals with an autosomal dominant inheritance. In most of these cases a mutation in the *CYLD* gene may be found, which is a tumor-suppressor gene located on chromosome 16q12–q13.[2–4] Different mutations in this gene have been reported to produce three distinct phenotypic variants. In multiple familial trichoepitheliomas (Online Mendelian Inheritance in Man [OMIM] 601,606), only multiple trichoepitheliomas can be found; in Brooke–Spiegler syndrome (OMIM 605,041), multiple trichoepitheliomas are associated with cylindromas and spiradenomas; in familial cylindromatosis (OMIM 132,700), which is the rarest condition, only multiple cylindromas are present (see Chapter 26).[5] On histopathologic examination, trichoepithelioma appears as a well-demarcated dermal tumor composed of nests of uniform basaloid (hair germ) cells, in which hair germ/papilla and bulbar differentiation are present. In addition, there are usually branching nests of basaloid cells and the presence of infundibulocystic structures. The stroma is loosely arranged and contains fibroblasts occasionally aggregated in abortive papillary-mesenchymal bodies.[6] The main differential diagnosis of trichoepithelioma involves basal cell carcinoma (BCC) and other adnexal tumors, in particular, trichoadenoma and trichoblastoma.[1]

DERMOSCOPY

In general, both solitary and multiple trichoepitheliomas are similar and frequently indistinguishable from BCC at dermoscopic examination. Indeed, both nonpigmented and pigmented BCC-specific criteria are frequently reported in trichoepithelioma.[7] In particular, blue-gray globules and blue-gray ovoid nests are the most frequently reported pigmented criteria (Figure 16.1a, b), while linear and/or branching on-focus vessels are the most frequently seen dermoscopic feature in both pigmented and nonpigmented forms (Figure 16.1c, d).[8] The presence of white structures has been suggested as a dermoscopic clue for distinguishing BCC from trichoepithelioma, as well as from other hair follicle tumors.[9] Specifically, in classic trichoepithelioma, a whitish background, shiny white areas and milia-like cysts have been described (Figure 16.1e, f).[10] Trichoepitheliomas associated with Brooke–Spiegler syndrome have the same dermoscopic features of the solitary form. In Figure 16.2 some amelanotic trichoepitheliomas are reported, located both on the face and the trunk. Linear and/or branching vessels could be identified; however, no white structures were present in the reported cases.

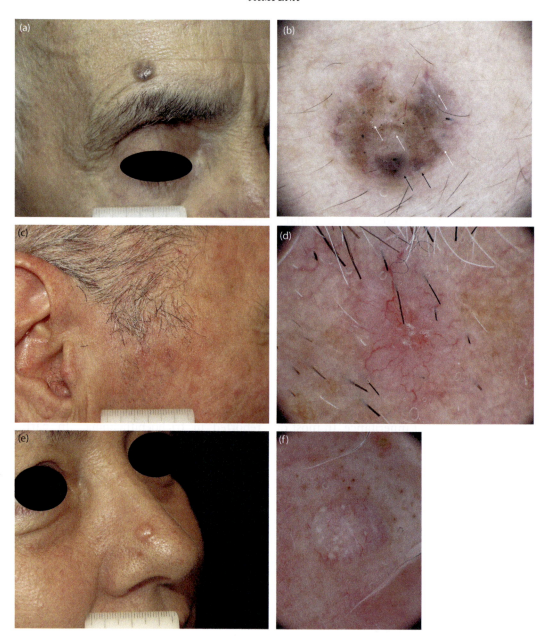

Figure 16.1 Solitary trichoepitheliomas located on the face: (a) clinical picture showing a 7-mm pigmented papule on the right eyebrow of an 82-year-old man; (b) corresponding dermoscopic image showing the presence of diffuse blue-gray globules and some blue-gray ovoid nests (black arrows) on a brownish background. Linear on-focus vessels, together with white streaks and milia-like cysts (white arrows), were also visible. (c) clinical picture revealing a 5-mm nonpigmented lesion on the preauricular right area of a 69-year-old man; (d) on dermoscopic examination, only on-focus linear and branching vessels on a whitish background were visible; (e) clinical appearance of a 6-mm flesh-colored papule located on the nose of a 54-year-old woman; (f) on dermoscopic appearance, on-focus branched vessels on a whitish background may be seen, together with white streaks and white circles diffuse through the lesion.

TRICHOEPITHELIOMA

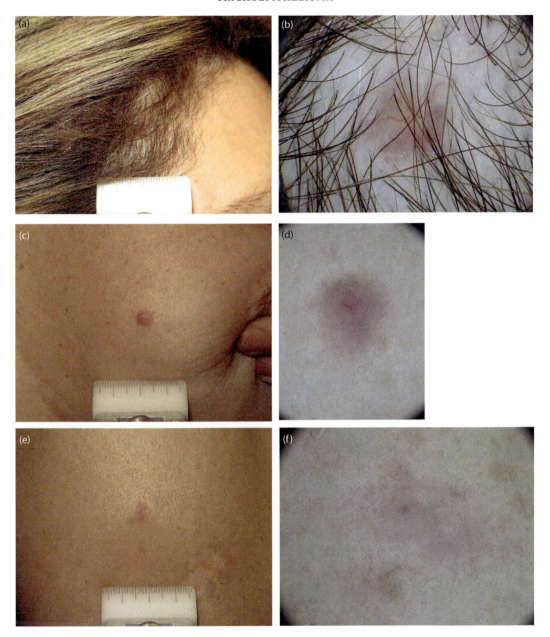

Figure 16.2 Clinical and dermoscopic pictures of amelanotic trichoepitheliomas in a 54-year-old woman affected by Brooke–Spiegler syndrome: (a, c, e) clinical pictures of 4–6 mm papules located on the right temple, breast and shoulder, respectively; (b, d, f) corresponding dermoscopic pictures revealing the presence of linear vessels on a pinkish background in all cases.

REFERENCES

1. Tellechea O, Cardoso JC, Reis JP, Ramos L, Gameiro AR, Coutinho I, Baptista AP. Benign follicular tumors. *An Bras Dermatol.* 2015;**90**(6):780–96; quiz 797–8.

2. Bowen S, Gill M, Lee DA et al. Mutations in the *CYLD* gene in Brooke-Spiegler syndrome, familial cylindromatosis, and multiple familial trichoepithelioma: Lack of genotype-phenotype correlation. *J Invest Dermatol.* 2005;**124**:919–20.

3. Young AL, Kellermayer R, Szigeti R et al. *CYLD* mutations underlie Brooke-Spiegler, familial cylindromatosis, and multiple familial trichoepithelioma syndromes. *Clin Genet.* 2006;**70**:246–9.
4. Saggar S, Chernoff KA, Lodha S et al. *CYLD* mutations in familial skin appendage tumours. *J Med Genet.* 2008;**45**:298–302.
5. Tellechea O, Reis JP, Freitas JD, Poiares Baptista A. Multiple eccrine spiradenoma and tricoepiteliomata. *Eur J Dermatol.* 1991;**1**:111–5.
6. Stanoszek LM, Wang GY, Harms PW. Histologic mimics of basal cell carcinoma. *Arch Pathol Lab Med.* 2017;**141**(11):1490–502.
7. Papageorgiou V, Apalla Z, Sotiriou E, Papageorgiou C, Lazaridou E, Vakirlis S, Ioannides D, Lallas A. The limitations of dermoscopy: False-positive and false-negative tumours. *J Eur Acad Dermatol Venereol.* 2018;**32**(6): 879–88.
8. Sgambato A, Zalaudek I, Ferrara G et al. Adnexal tumors: Clinical and dermoscopic mimickers of basal cell carcinoma. *Arch Dermatol.* 2008;**144**:426.
9. Lallas A, Moscarella E, Argenziano G, Longo C, Apalla Z, Ferrara G, Piana S, Rosato S, Zalaudek I. Dermoscopy of uncommon skin tumours. *Australas J Dermatol.* 2014;**55**(1):53–62.
10. Navarrete-Dechent C, Bajaj S, Marghoob AA, González S, Muñoz D. Multiple familial trichoepithelioma: Confirmation via dermoscopy. *Dermatol Pract Concept.* 2016;**6**(3):51–4.

17 Desmoplastic trichoepithelioma

Riccardo Pampena

INTRODUCTION

Desmoplastic trichoepithelioma (DTE) is a variant of trichoepithelioma with specific clinicopathologic features. It occurs almost exclusively on the face of young adult women, in particular on the forehead and malar regions.

Desmoplastic trichoepithelioma generally appears as a solitary, hard, small plaque of 5 mm in diameter, with raised borders and a depressed center, which gives an annular appearance. Occasionally, lesions are multiple.[1] On histopathologic examination, DTE appears

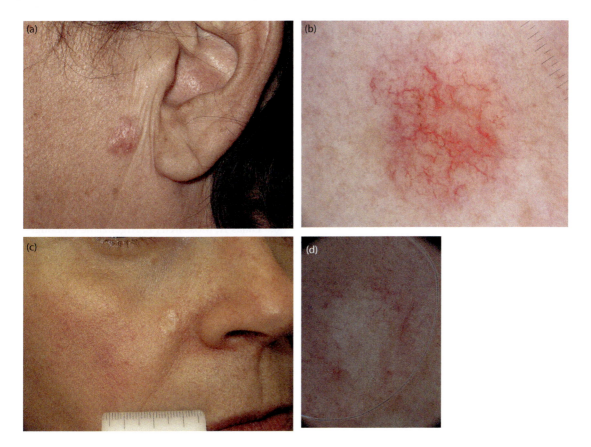

Figure 17.1 Clinical and dermoscopic pictures of two cases of desmoplastic trichoepitheliomas with a plaque-like appearance: (a) the first lesion was located on the left preauricular region of a 56-year-old woman, was 8 mm in diameter and displayed a pinkish homogenous color; (b) on dermoscopic examination, it was characterized by a pinkish background and linear/branched in-focus vessels; (c) the second lesion was located on the right cheek of a 55-year-old woman, was 6 mm in diameter and was characterized by a whitish appearance and a depressed center; (d) on dermoscopic examination, some linear in-focus vessels may be seen on a whitish background. Some milia-like cysts were also visible in the central part of the lesion.

as a dermal well-circumscribed lesion with a central depression. The tumor is made of irregular cords and small nests of basaloid cells and keratinous cysts, which are frequently calcified. Atypical mitoses and cytologic atypia are absent. An abundant, dense and hypocellular desmoplastic stroma surrounds these epithelial structures.[2]

The main differential diagnosis on histopathologic examination is morpheaform basal cell carcinoma (BCC). Differently from BCC, DTE does not display clefting between the tumor and the stroma but between the stroma and the adjacent dermis, and it has more infundibulocystic differentiation; necrosis and mitoses are generally absent, and CK20/Cam 5.2-positive cells are often seen, which correspond to Merkel cells.[3]

DERMOSCOPY

Even on dermoscopic examination, the main differential diagnosis of DTE is represented by morpheaform BCC. DTE commonly displays BCC-specific criteria, in particular in-focus linear or arborizing vessels, but also pigmented criteria such as multiple blue-gray globules and large blue-gray ovoid nests (Figure 17.1a, b). Both of these tumors are characterized by a whitish background color; however, in morpheaform BCC it generally has a scar-like appearance, whereas in DTE, a typical ivory hue has been described. Other white structures, such as milia-like cysts, may also be seen in DTE and correspond to keratinous cysts (Figure 17.1c, d).[4-6]

REFERENCES

1. Brownstein MH, Shapiro L. Desmoplastic trichoepithelioma. *Cancer*. 1977;**40**:2979–86.
2. Tellechea O, Cardoso JC, Reis JP, Ramos L, Gameiro AR, Coutinho I, Baptista AP. Benign follicular tumors. *An Bras Dermatol*. 2015;**90**(6):780–96; quiz 797–8.
3. Wang Q, Ghimire D, Wang J, Luo S, Li Z, Wang H, Geng S, Xiao S, Zheng Y. Desmoplastic trichoepithelioma: A clinicopathological study of three cases and a review of the literature. *Oncol Lett*. 2015;**10**(4):2468–76.
4. Papageorgiou V, Apalla Z, Sotiriou E, Papageorgiou C, Lazaridou E, Vakirlis S, Ioannides D, Lallas A. The limitations of dermoscopy: False-positive and false-negative tumours. *J Eur Acad Dermatol Venereol*. 2018;**32**(6):879–88.
5. Khelifa E, Masouyé I, Kaya G, Le Gal FA. Dermoscopy of desmoplastic trichoepithelioma reveals other criteria to distinguish it from basal cell carcinoma. *Dermatology*. 2013;**226**(2):101–4.
6. Lallas A, Moscarella E, Argenziano G, Longo C, Apalla Z, Ferrara G, Piana S, Rosato S, Zalaudek I. Dermoscopy of uncommon skin tumours. *Australas J Dermatol*. 2014;**55**(1):53–62.

18 Trichoblastoma

Riccardo Pampena

INTRODUCTION

Trichoblastoma is a rare benign tumor of the hair germ, mainly composed of follicular germinative cells. Together with the syringocystadenoma papilliferum, it is the most common benign tumor arising in organoid (sebaceous) nevus.[1] Clinically, it generally appears as a slow-growing nodule of the head and neck, greater than 1 cm in diameter. Several variants of trichoblastoma have been described, including pigmented, giant, clear cell and adamantanoid. Of note, trichoepithelioma could represent a superficial (intradermal) and differentiated variant of trichoblastoma.[2]

On histopathologic examination, it appears as a well-circumscribed, symmetric dermal-hypodermal tumor composed of irregular

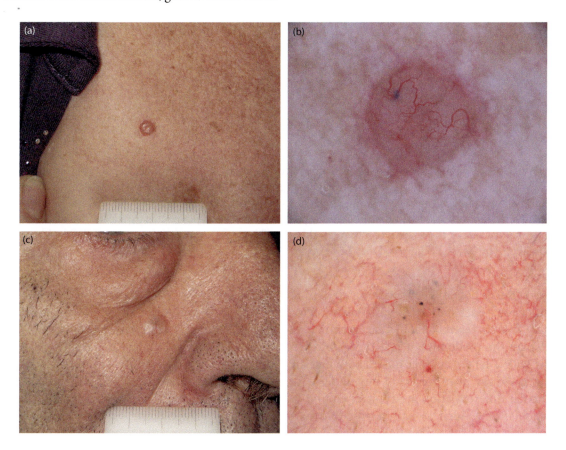

Figure 18.1 Clinical and dermoscopic pictures of four cases of trichoblastoma: (a, c) the first and the second cases consisted of two papular amelanotic lesions, of 4–5 mm in diameter, located on the breast area of a 63-year-old woman and on the right cheek of a 77-year-old man; (b, d) on dermoscopic examination, both of these lesions displayed on-focus linear and arborizing vessels on a pinkish (first lesion) and whitish (second lesion) background. One and multiple blue-gray globules could also be seen, respectively. *(Continued)*

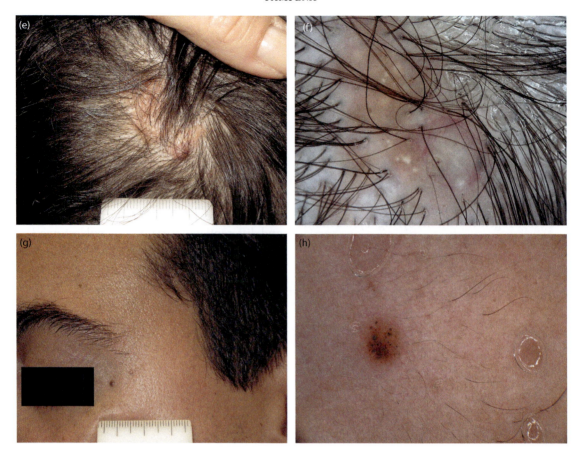

Figure 18.1 (*Continued*) Clinical and dermoscopic pictures of four cases of trichoblastoma: (e) clinical picture of a flesh-colored papule arising in the context of an organoid nevus located on the vertex area of a 26-year-old man; (f) on dermoscopy, linear vessels and a blue-gray ovoid nest may be seen on a white-pinkish background, together with several milia-like cysts; (g) clinical appearance of a small pigmented papule located on the external periocular area of the left eye of a 33-year-old man; (h) on dermoscopic examination, diffuse blue-gray globules on a brownish background may be seen.

nests of small basaloid cells with no epidermal connection. Basaloid cells with scant cytoplasm, which resemble follicular germinative cells, are the predominant cell type; however, cells with a larger cytoplasm, resembling hair stem cells, are also present. Limited signs of follicular differentiation are typically found in trichoblastoma, such as hair papilla and hair germ formation. An abundant dense or cellular stroma surrounds the epithelial structures. Differently from basal cell carcinoma (BCC), clefts are present between the stroma and the dermis, and not between the stroma and the epithelial structures; also, mitoses and cytologic atypia are typically absent, as is necrosis.[3] The principal differential diagnosis of trichoblastoma is represented by BCC. On histopathologic examination, the aforementioned criteria are generally sufficient to differentiate these tumors; however, on clinical and dermoscopic examination, the differential diagnosis is frequently impossible.[4]

DERMOSCOPY

No specific dermoscopic features of trichoblastoma have been described so far, allowing the differentiation of this entity from BCC.

One study comparing the dermoscopic aspect a of trichoblastoma and trichoblastic BCC[5] showed that the former more frequently displayed arborizing vessels and spoke-wheel areas, while blue-ovoid nests mainly characterized trichoblastic BCC. Authors concluded that no specific dermoscopic criteria allowed for differentiation of trichoblastoma from BCC (Figure 18.1a–f). Concerning trichoblastoma arising in a nevus sebaceous, Zaballos and colleagues reported in 2015[1] a series of 23 cases that were mainly characterized by a symmetric shape and a blue-gray homogenous area occupying the whole lesion (total large blue-gray ovoid nest). Other frequently seen dermoscopic features were arborizing and small fine vessels and white structures, while large blue-gray ovoid nests and multiple blue-gray globules only characterized a minority of lesions, as compared to BCC (Figure 18.1g, h).

REFERENCES

1. Zaballos P, Serrano P, Flores G et al. Dermoscopy of tumours arising in naevus sebaceous: A morphological study of 58 cases. *J Eur Acad Dermatol Venereol.* 2015;**29**(11):2231–7.
2. Tellechea O, Cardoso JC, Reis JP, Ramos L, Gameiro AR, Coutinho I, Baptista AP. Benign follicular tumors. *An Bras Dermatol.* 2015;**90**(6):780–96; quiz 797–8.
3. Papageorgiou V, Apalla Z, Sotiriou E, Papageorgiou C, Lazaridou E, Vakirlis S, Ioannides D, Lallas A. The limitations of dermoscopy: False-positive and false-negative tumours. *J Eur Acad Dermatol Venereol.* 2018;**32**(6):879–88.
4. Lallas A, Moscarella E, Argenziano G, Longo C, Apalla Z, Ferrara G, Piana S, Rosato S, Zalaudek I. Dermoscopy of uncommon skin tumours. *Australas J Dermatol.* 2014;**55**(1):53–62.
5. Ghigliotti G, De Col E, Parodi A, Bombonato C, Argenziano G. Trichoblastoma: Is a clinical or dermoscopic diagnosis possible? *J Eur Acad Dermatol Venereol.* 2016;**30**(11):1978–80.

19 Tumors of the follicular infundibulum

Riccardo Pampena

INTRODUCTION

Despite its name, a tumor of the follicular infundibulum (infundibuloma) actually originates from the isthmic part of the hair follicle.[1] A real infundibular origin is only seen with two other adnexal tumors: inverted follicular keratosis and dilatated pore of Winer. The latter is a quite common lesion and is not discussed in this book. Both the tumor of the follicular infundibulum and the inverted follicular keratosis generally appear on the head and neck area of elderly patients as a solitary papule, with a smooth or keratotic surface.[2] Some clinical variants of the tumor of the follicular infundibulum have been described, such as eruptive infundibulomatosis and multiple hypopigmented lesions. Histopathologically it appears as a plate-like subepidermal tumor composed of interconnected strands of pale glycogen-containing keratinocytes, which are also connected to the epidermis and to follicular structures.[3] Concerning the inverted follicular keratosis, three clinical variants have been reported: flesh-colored nodular, papillomatous and keratoacanthoma-like. On histopathologic examination, the inverted follicular keratosis is instead characterized by an endophytic appearance with large lobules or finger-like projections into the surrounding dermis. Each lobule is composed of basaloid cells at the periphery and squamous cells in the central part.[4] The differential diagnosis of these tumors is broad, including basal cell carcinoma, keratoacanthoma, squamous cell carcinoma, seborrheic keratosis, viral warts and other adnexal tumors.[1]

DERMOSCOPY

In 2016, Llambrich and colleagues described the dermoscopic aspects of a series of 12

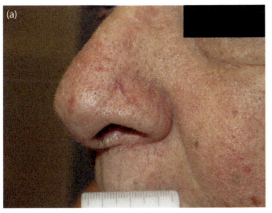
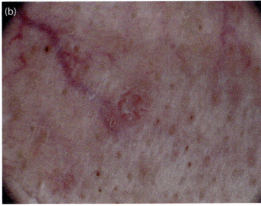

Figure 19.1 Clinical and dermoscopic pictures of a 71-year-old woman with an inverted follicular keratosis located on the left side of her nose: (a) on clinical examination a small (2 mm in diameter) reddish and whitish papule may be seen; (b) dermoscopically some structureless whitish areas intermingled with linear/branching vessels are visible, which are mainly located at the periphery of the lesion.

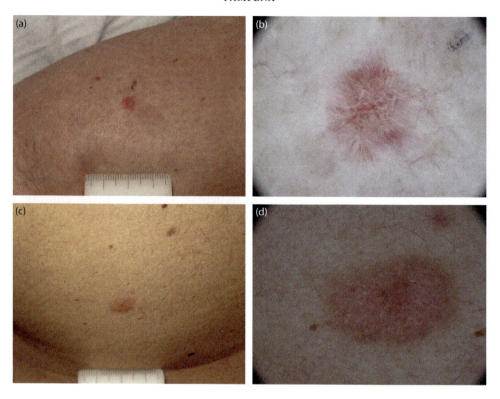

Figure 19.2 Clinical and dermoscopic pictures of two cases of tumor of the follicular infundibulum: (a) the first lesion was flat and amelanotic and was located on the lower limbs of a 54-year-old woman; (b) an appearance resembling dermatofibroma or basal cell carcinoma could be recognized on dermoscopic examination, with the presence of short in-focus linear vessels at the periphery and more convoluted vessels in the central part, together with the presence of short shiny whitish lines; (c) the second lesion was flat and amelanotic and located on the back of a 52-year-old man; (d) dermoscopically it was characterized by dotted vessels and negative pigmented network, together with a brownish background, giving an overall melanoma-like appearance.

inverted follicular keratosis.[5] They found that specific white structures were present in all of the cases, in particular, scales and structureless areas. In addition, vascular structures were always present, with the most reported being hairpin vessels with white halo, seen in a radial arrangement. Keratin was present in most cases and was often located in the central areas of the lesion. Most of the lesions displayed a keratoacanthoma-like appearance (Figure 19.1). No cases have been published so far reporting the dermoscopic aspect of the tumor of the follicular infundibulum. By reviewing our database, we retrieved clinical and dermoscopic pictures of two cases that were characterized on dermoscopic examination by different combinations of criteria, such as in-focus linear and arborizing vessels, more convoluted vessels, central ulceration and a negative pigmented network (Figure 19.2). As shown by these two cases, a tumor of the follicular infundibulum may be a great simulator on a clinical and dermoscopic basis, and histopathologic examination is needed to make the final diagnosis.

REFERENCES

1. Ackerman AB, Viragh PA, Chongchitnant N. *Neoplasms with Follicular Differentiation.* Philadelphia, PA: Lea & Febiger; 1993:553.

2. Alomari A, Subtil A, Owen CE, McNiff JM. Solitary and multiple tumors of follicular infundibulum: A review of 168 cases with emphasis on staining patterns and clinical variants. *J Cutan Pathol.* 2013;**40**(6):532–7.
3. Cribier B, Grosshans E. Tumor of the follicular infundibulum: A clinicopathologic study. *J Am Acad Dermatol.* 1995;**33**:979.
4. Battistella M, Peltre B, Cribier B. Composite tumors associating trichoblastoma and benign epidermal/follicular neoplasm: Another proof of the follicular nature of inverted follicular keratosis. *J Cutan Pathol.* 2010;**37**(10):1057–63.
5. Llambrich A, Zaballos P, Taberner R, Terrasa F, Bañuls J, Pizarro A, Malvehy J, Puig S. Dermoscopy of inverted follicular keratosis: Study of 12 cases. *Clin Exp Dermatol.* 2016;**41**(5):468–73.

20 Tricholemmoma and tricholemmal carcinoma and Cowden syndrome

Eugenia Veronica Di Brizzi, Simonetta Piana, Giuseppe Argenziano, and Elvira Moscarella

INTRODUCTION

Tricholemmoma is a benign tumor with differentiation toward pilosebaceous follicular epithelium. Tricholemmal carcinoma is the malignant form of tricholemmoma with outer root sheath differentiation. Both tumors were described first by Headington and French in 1962.[1]

Tricholemmoma occurs in all races and both sexes. Clinically, it presents as solitary or multiple keratotic, flesh-topped and small papules (usually less than 5 mm), generally located on the face, nose, eyelids and lips[2] and can mimic a basal cell carcinoma, squamous cell carcinoma or wart.[3]

Multiple facial tricholemmomas are often associated with Cowden syndrome, a rare autosomal dominant genodermatosis caused by mutation in the *PTEN* gene characterized by hamartomatous intestinal polyps, breast or other visceral cancers and skin tumors such as hamartomas and adnexal tumor.[4] Recognition of these skin tumors could determine a diagnosis of this rare syndrome.

Histologically, tricholemmoma is a sharply circumscribed lobulated neoplasm composed of a prominent palisade of uniform cuboidal to columnar periodic acid–Schiff (PAS) positive cells, showing variable glycogen vacuolation, which extend into the upper dermis, usually in continuity with the epidermis or with follicular epithelium at several points. The peripheral layer of columnar cells with nuclear palisading resembles the outer root sheath of hair follicles.[5]

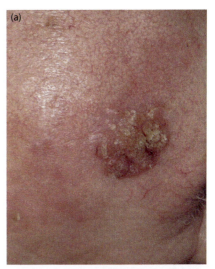

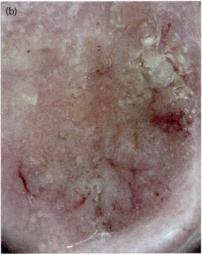

Figure 20.1 Clinical and dermoscopic features of a tricholemmoma arising on the frontal area of an 88-year-old man. (a) The lesion is nonpigmented and has a verrucous surface. (b) In dermoscopy, keratin masses and perivascular whitish halos are seen.

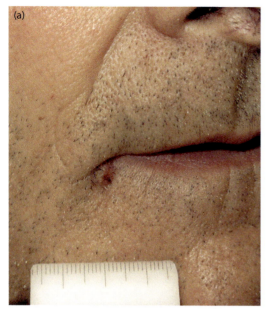

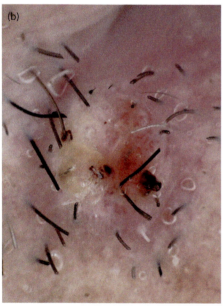

Figure 20.2 (a) A tricholemmoma in a 65-year-old man. The lesion is an ulcerated nonpigmented nodule of the face. (b) In dermoscopy, white and yellow areas, linear vessels and a central crust are seen.

DERMOSCOPY

Dermoscopically, this tumor shows a radiated area with erythematous radial lines surrounded by white shiny areas, several lesions show a hyperpigmented halo, which may possibly

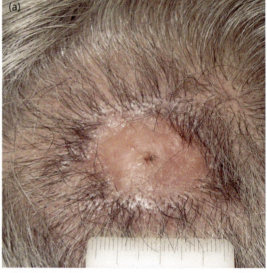

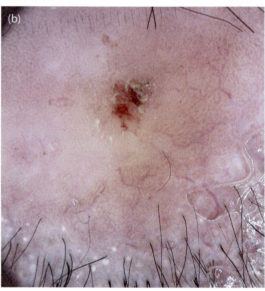

Figure 20.3 (a) A tricholemmal carcinoma resembling an area of cicatricial alopecia, on the scalp of a 77-year-old man. (b) In dermoscopy, few linear vessels are visible over a white-yellowish background.

represent secondary hyperpigmentation due to persistent scratching.[5]

Several treatment options are reported. In solitary lesions, surgical excision is recommended because it can simulate malignant tumors. Carbon dioxide laser is particularly useful if a patient presents with multiple tricholemmomas (Figures 20.1 and 20.2).[6]

Tricholemmal carcinoma occurs most commonly on the face, scalp or neck of the elderly as an asymptomatic exophytic or polypoid mass, sometimes associated with ulceration, scales and telangiectasia, or as an alopecic area. It is generally about 2 cm in diameter.[7,8]

Unlike the tricholemmoma, very few cases have been described in association with the Cowden syndrome.[8]

Differential diagnosis includes basal cell carcinoma, squamous cell carcinoma, keratoacanthoma or proliferating pilar cyst.[8,9] Histopathologic examination shows features similar to tricholemmoma but with cellular atypia and a high mitotic index.[1] The growth is lobular, infiltrative and often centered on a pilosebaceous unit. In the center of the tumor the cells are polygonal, large and clear PAS positive, with glycogen in cytoplasm. The cells at the periphery are often palisaded, and sometimes pagetoid spread can be seen.[8]

Dermoscopically, tricholemmal carcinoma shows a polymorphous vascular pattern, consisting of dotted, linear, irregular and tortuous vessels, in conjunction with white-yellowish well-circumscribed areas and ulceration (Figure 20.3).[10]

Regarding the therapy, surgical excision is recommended, and local recurrence was reported in a few cases. Other therapeutic options are cryotherapy and imiquimod 5% cream.[8]

REFERENCES

1. Headington JT. Tumors of the hair follicle. A Review. *Am J Pathol.* 1976;**85**:479–514.
2. Divya S, Taylor RS. Appendage tumors and hamartomas of the skin. In: Goldsmith LA, Katz SI, Gilchrest BA, Paller AS, Leffell DJ, Wolff K, eds. *Fitzpatrick's Dermatology in General Medicine*, 8th ed. New York, NY: McGraw-Hill Medical; 2012:1337–62.
3. Reifler DM, Ballitch HA, Kessler DL et al. Tricholemmoma of the eyelid. *Ophthalmology.* 1987;**94**(10):1272–5.
4. Brownstein MH, Mehregan AH, Bikowski JB. Trichilemmomas in Cowden's disease. *JAMA.* 1977;**238**(1):26–32.
5. Horcajada-Reales C, Avilés-Izquierdo JA, Ciudad-Blanco C et al. Dermoscopic pattern in facial trichilemmomas: Red iris-like structure. *J Am Acad Dermatol.* 2015;**72**(1 Suppl):S30–2.
6. Chang IK, Lee Y, Seo YJ et al. Treatment of multiple trichilemmomas with the pinhole method using a carbon dioxide laser in a patient with Cowden syndrome. *Dermatol Ther.* 2015;**28**(2):71–3.
7. Reis JP, Tellechea O, Cunha MF, Baptista AP. Trichilemmal carcinoma: Review of 8 cases. *J Cutan Pathol.* 1993;**20**:44–9.
8. Hamman MS, Brian Jiang SI. Management of trichilemmal carcinoma: An update and comprehensive review of the literature. *Dermatol Surg.* 2014;**40**(7):711–7.
9. Boscaino A, Terracciano LM, Donofrio V, et al. Tricholemmal carcinoma: A study of seven cases. *J Cutan Pathol.* 1992;**19**:94–9.
10. Lallas A, Moscarella E, Argenziano G et al. Dermoscopy of uncommon skin tumours. *Australas J Dermatol.* 2014;**55**(1):53–62.

21 Pilomatrixoma

Riccardo Pampena

INTRODUCTION

Even if uncommon, pilomatrixoma represents the most common benign adnexal skin tumor with a peak in pediatric ages and a smaller one in the sixth decade.[1] It shows a differentiation toward the matrix of the hair follicle and is characteristically firm to hard at palpation, depending on the amount of calcification. Pilomatrixoma, also called pilomatricoma or calcifying epithelioma of Malherbe, generally appears as a solitary derma-hypodermal nodule, from 0.5 to 3.0 cm in diameter, located on the head and neck region or on the upper limbs. Clinically, a combination of gray, brown and white areas is frequently seen. Occasionally it can be multiple, especially in patients with Gardner's syndrome or myotonic muscular dystrophy.[2] Concerning pathogenesis, a dysregulation of the WNT/β-catenin pathway has been reported in most cases of pilomatrixoma.[3]

On histopathologic examination, it generally appears as a well-circumscribed derma-hypodermal nodule surrounded by a pseudocapsule. Two cellular types of epithelial origin can be found, whose relative proportion varies according to the age of the lesion. In most recent tumors, small basophilic cells with scant cytoplasm (matrical cells) predominate and are generally located in the peripheral part; in older lesions, however, cells without the nucleus and with abundant eosinophilic cytoplasm (ghost cells) predominate. These are commonly located in the central part of the tumor and correspond to terminal differentiation of the matrical cells. In addition, in older lesions foci of calcification are commonly seen.[4] A wide range of possible differential diagnoses should be considered, such as hemangioma, cyst, lipoma, basal cell carcinoma, squamous cell carcinoma and melanocytic lesions.[5]

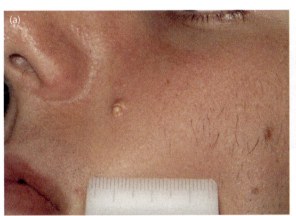 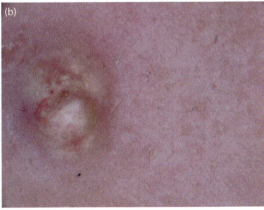

Figure 21.1 Clinical and dermoscopic images of four cases of pilomatrixoma: (a) the first lesion was located on the left cheek of a 16-year-old young man. It clinically appeared as a 4 mm whitish and firm polylobate papule; (b) on dermoscopic examination a white-brownish background may be seen with some linear irregular vessels.

(Continued)

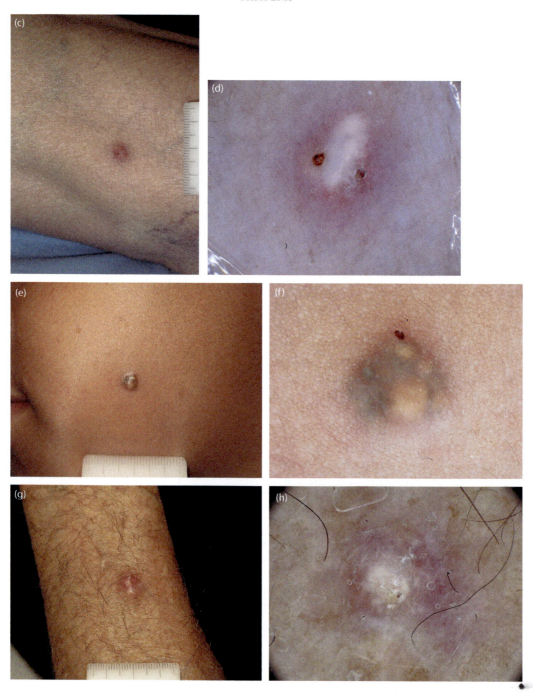

Figure 21.1 (Continued) Clinical and dermoscopic images of four cases of pilomatrixoma: (c) the second case was located on the left thigh of a 79-year-old woman and appeared as a 5 mm pinkish firm papule; (d) on dermoscopy a central whitish area may be seen with two small ulcerations and some linear-irregular vessels in the peripheral part; (e) the third lesion was located on the left cheek of an 11-year-old young man and was clinically characterized by a whitish nodule firm at palpation, with a peripheral pigmented part; (f) on dermoscopic examination multiple yellowish areas intermingled with some bluish areas may be seen, together with a small ulceration in the upper part; (g) the fourth lesions consisted of a 0.9 mm amelanotic papule on the left arm of an 85-year-old man, firm at palpation; (h) dermoscopically it was characterized by a central whitish area and a peripheral pinkish area.

DERMOSCOPY

The largest series of pilomatricoma evaluated by dermoscopy was published in 2008 by Zaballos et al.[6] and consisted of 10 cases located on the head and neck and upper extremities. Authors reported that a diagnosis of pilomatricoma was considered in only half of the cases on a clinical basis, while in nine cases using the dermoscope. Concerning the dermoscopic features, irregular whitish structures and streaks were present in the majority of cases, together with some vascular structures: reddish homogenous areas, hairpin and linear-irregular vessels; besides, ulceration and blue-gray areas were also reported. Interestingly, specific criteria for melanocytic and nonmelanocytic tumors were absent in all cases. Whitish structures were histopathologically correlated to the presence of calcification or keratin masses within the tumor. Other reports indicated irregular white and/or yellow structures, reddish homogenous areas, linear vessels and white streaks as the most frequently seen dermoscopic features in pilomatrixoma (Figure 21.1).[7–9]

REFERENCES

1. Julian CG, Bowers PW. A clinical review of 209 pilomatricomas. *J Am Acad Dermatol*. 1998;**39**:191–5.
2. Marrogi AJ, Wick MR, Dehner LP. Pilomatrical neoplasms in children and young adults. *Am J Dermatopathol*. 1992;**14**:87–94.
3. Chan EF, Gat U, McNiff JM, Fuchs E. A common human skin tumour is caused by activating mutations in ß-catenin. *Nat Genet*. 1999;**21**:410–3.
4. Herrmann JL, Allan A, Trapp KM, Morgan MB. Pilomatrix carcinoma: 13 new cases and review of the literature with emphasis in predictors of metastasis. *J Am Acad Dermatol*. 2014;**71**:38–43.e2.
5. Tellechea O, Cardoso JC, Reis JP, Ramos L, Gameiro AR, Coutinho I, Baptista AP. Benign follicular tumors. *An Bras Dermatol*. 2015;**90**(6):780–96; quiz 797–8.
6. Zaballos P, Llambrich A, Puig S, Malvehy J. Dermoscopic findings of pilomatricomas. *Dermatology*. 2008;**217**(3):225–30.
7. Barreto-Chang OL, Gorell ES, Yamaguma MA et al. Diagnosis of pilomatricoma using an otoscope. *Pediatr Dermatol*. 2010;**27**:554–7.
8. Ayhan E, Ertugay O, Gundogdu R. Three different dermoscopic views of three new cases with pilomatrixoma. *Int J Trichology*. 2014;**6**(1):21–2.
9. Lallas A, Moscarella E, Argenziano G, Longo C, Apalla Z, Ferrara G, Piana S, Rosato S, Zalaudek I. Dermoscopy of uncommon skin tumours. *Australas J Dermatol*. 2014;**55**(1):53–62.

22 Fibrofolliculoma/trichodiscoma and Birt–Hogg–Dubè syndrome

Giovanni Paolino and Elvira Moscarella

INTRODUCTION

Among uncommon tumors, fibrofolliculomas (FFs) and trichodiscomas (TDs) play a pivotal role, since they are a hallmark of the rare Birt–Hogg–Dubè syndrome (BHDS).

BHDS is an autosomal dominant form of genodermatosis caused by germline mutations in the folliculin (*FLCN*) gene, which is mapped to the p11.2 region, in chromosome 17.[1] BHDS is commonly characterized by pulmonary cysts, renal cell carcinoma, recurrent pneumothoraxes and multiple FFs/TDs, mainly disposed in the head and neck region.[1] Accordingly, prompt recognition of the cutaneous manifestations is critical for a correct diagnosis of BHDS; for this reason, the dermatologic criterion of "five or more facial or truncal papules, of which at least one was confirmed histologically as FF or TD" should always be utilized.[2,3] To date, the presence of multiple cutaneous lesions remains a major criterion for the diagnosis of BHDS, and the diagnosis can be made even when an *FCLN* genetic test is negative.[1]

Also in these rare forms of tumors, dermoscopy could be used as a valid and additional diagnostic method for clinicians. In a case series, Jarrett et al. described FF as dermoscopically characterized by the presence of well-demarcated areas of pallor with central follicular openings.[4]

To date, both FF and TD are considered to be hamartomas that develop from the mantle cells of the infundibular portion of hair follicles and surrounding connective tissues.[2,5] Histologically, FF is mainly characterized by the immature structure of hair follicles, with a mantle-like proliferation of epithelial strands

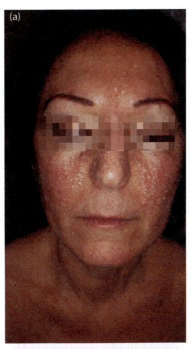

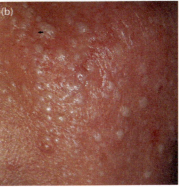

Figure 22.1 (a) A 62-year-old Caucasian female patient, with a 5-year history of asymptomatic, multiple facial papules, showing a uniform whitish-ivory color. The lesions histologically corresponded with fibrofolliculoma (FF). (b) Detail of the lesions in Figure 22.1a. Note the presence of the follicular openings (black arrow). *(Continued)*

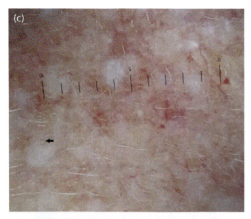
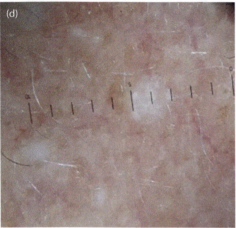

Figure 22.1 (Continued) (c) Dermoscopy shows papular lesions with a homogeneous whitish pattern and with the typical follicular openings (see black arrow). (d) Dermoscopy of other lesions highlights how the dermoscopic patterns are repetitive, showing always the same features.

from the infundibular part of the hair follicles.[2] The stroma surrounding the epithelium is densely fibrous and sclerotic and may contain mucin. While in FF there is a predominance of the epithelium component, in TD there is a predominance of the connective component. Specifically, in TD there is often a folliculosebaceous collarette surrounding the fibroblastic proliferation, the stroma is more fibrous than FF and there is a disappearance of the mantle-like proliferation of epithelial strands.[2] For both FF and TD the main histologic differential diagnoses are basal cell carcinoma, neurofollicular hamartoma and perifollicular fibroma.

Recently, a newly described cutaneous lesion was reported, associated with BHDS, the "angiomatous nodules." These are skin angiomatous lesions with prominent signet-ring features in histology. Clinically, they appear as small papules, translucent and with neat borders being in differential diagnosis with acrochordon. On dermoscopic examination, light brown structureless areas with tiny not-in-focus vessels were observed.[6]

Regarding the therapy of FF and TD, no further treatments are necessary once the diagnosis is reached, except for aesthetic reasons. In any case, the main treatments are surgery, cryotherapy and laser.

DERMOSCOPY

To date, only one report described the dermoscopic features of FF in the context of BHDS.[4] Jarrett et al. described FF as characterized by the presence of well-demarcated areas of pallor with central follicular openings.[4] Following is reported the case of a 62-year-old Caucasian female patient with a 5-year history of asymptomatic, multiple facial papules, showing a uniform whitish-ivory color (Figure 22.1a, b). Four years before, the patient removed a renal cell carcinoma, in her right kidney. On dermoscopic examination, the lesions showed a homogeneous whitish pattern, with the presence of characteristic follicular openings (Figure 22.1c, d). A biopsy of one of the facial lesions confirmed the diagnosis of FF, and a diagnosis of BHDS was performed. At the clinic-pathologic correlation, the whitish dermoscopic features of FF correspond with the dense fibrosis present in the stroma of the tumor, while the follicular openings correspond with the mantle-like proliferation of epithelial strands from the infundibular port of the hair follicles.

REFERENCES

1. Hao S, Long F, Sun F, Liu T, Li D, Jiang S. Birt-Hogg-Dubé syndrome: A literature review and case study of a Chinese woman presenting a novel FLCN mutation. *BMC Pulm Med*. 2017;**17**:43.

2. Iwabuchi C, Ebana H, Ishiko A, Negishi A, Mizobuchi T, Kumasaka T, Kurihara M, Seyama K. Skin lesions of Birt-Hogg-Dubé syndrome: Clinical and histopathological findings in 31 Japanese patients who presented with pneumothorax and/or multiple lung cysts. *J Dermatol Sci.* 2018;**89**(1):77–84.
3. Toro JR, Glenn G, Duray P, Darling T, Weirich G, Zbar B, Linehan M, Turner ML. Birt-Hogg-Dubé syndrome: A novel marker of kidney neoplasia. *Arch Dermatol.* 1999;**135**:1195–202.
4. Jarrett R, Walker L, Side L, Bowling J. Dermoscopic features of Birt-Hogg-Dubé syndrome. *Arch Dermatol.* 2009;**145**:1208.
5. Ackerman AB, De Viragh P, Chongchitnant N. Fibrofolliculoma and trichodiscoma. In: Ackerman AB, De Viragh P, Chongchitnant N, eds. *Neoplasms with Follicular Differentiation.* Philadelphia, PA: Lea & Febiger; 1993:245–79.
6. Nikolaidou C, Moscarella E, Longo C, Rosato S, Cavazza A, Piana S. Multiple angiomatous nodules: A novel skin tumor in Birt-Hogg-Dubé syndrome. *J Cutan Pathol.* 2016;**43**(12):1197–202.

23 Sebaceous tumors

Riccardo Pampena

INTRODUCTION

Sebaceous tumors are uncommon entities that include sebaceous adenoma, sebaceoma (sebaceous epithelioma) and sebaceous carcinoma.[1,2] Sebaceous adenoma and sebaceoma are very similar at clinical presentation, appearing as slow-growing, flesh-colored solitary papules, mainly located on the head and neck region and generally involving elderly patients. Multiple forms in younger individuals are commonly seen in the context of the Muir–Torre syndrome. Multiple sebaceous carcinomas may also be seen in patients with Muir–Torre syndrome. Generally, this malignant tumor involves the ocular adnexa, particularly the meibomian and Zeis glands. Less commonly extraocular sites are involved; in these cases, sebaceous carcinoma appears as a yellowish firm papule, from 1 to 4 cm in diameter, often ulcerated and is more frequently seen on the head and neck of elderly patients.[3] On histopathologic examination, sebaceous adenoma appears as a dermal mass composed by sebaceous lobules separated by connective tissue septa. Darker germinative cells may be seen at the periphery of the lobules while paler mature cells are located in the central part. In sebaceoma multiple dermal nests are instead commonly seen, which are mainly composed of small basaloid cells with some mature sebaceous cells. Concerning sebaceous carcinoma, sheets or lobules of cells are commonly seen, which extend from the dermis to the subcutis and even to the underlying muscle.[4] Muir–Torre syndrome (Online Mendelian Inheritance in Man [OMIM] 158320) is an autosomal dominant disease and represents an allelic variant (accounting for 1%–2% of cases) of the hereditary nonpolyposis colon syndrome (Lynch syndrome). Mutations in some DNA mismatch repair genes have been demonstrated to cause Muir–Torre syndrome, being MSH2, MLH1 and MSH6 the most implicated. Mutations in these genes are associated with microsatellite instability that characterizes tumors associated with this syndrome. Muir–Torre syndrome is characterized by the development of sebaceous tumors in association with visceral neoplasms, most commonly gastrointestinal carcinomas. Other cutaneous findings may be keratoacanthomas and epidermal cysts. When sebaceous tumors are multiple and/or occur before the age of 50 years, Muir–Torre syndrome should always be suspected.[5]

DERMOSCOPY

Generally, differentiating among different types of sebaceous tumors is troublesome both clinically and dermoscopically. On dermoscopic examination, the combination of unfocused arborizing vessels and yellow structures is suggestive of sebaceous tumors. In particular, for sebaceous adenoma and sebaceoma two possible patterns have been described, with and without a central crater (Figure 23.1). In the first case, crown vessels are commonly seen surrounding a central opaque whitish structure; in cases without a central crater a whitish-yellow background with unfocused arborizing vessels and few yellow comedo-like structures have been described.[6–8] Concerning sebaceous carcinoma a homogenous yellowish background is commonly found, together with a polymorphous vascular pattern and ulceration (Figure 23.2).[9] The

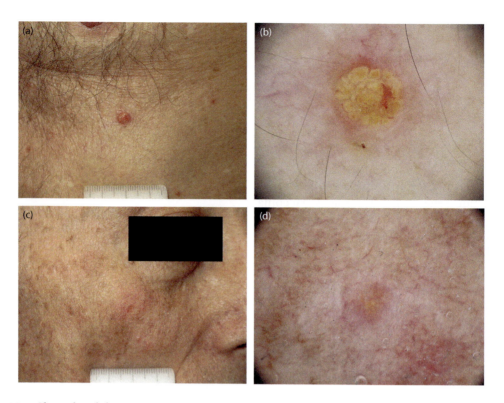

Figure 23.1 Clinical and dermoscopic images of benign sebaceous tumors: (a) clinical image of a sebaceous adenoma located on the chest of a 76-year-old man affected by Muir–Torre syndrome, which appears as a 5 mm yellowish papule; (b) at dermoscopic examination unfocused yellowish polygonal structures in the central part and unfocused vessels at the periphery of the lesion may be seen (pattern without a central crater); (c) clinical image of a sebaceoma located on the right cheek of the same patient, which appears as a 3 mm flesh-colored papule; (d) at dermoscopic examination a small central crater filled with yellowish amorphous material may be seen, surrounded by unfocused linear vessels.

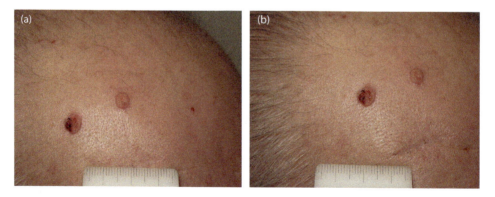

Figure 23.2 Clinical and dermoscopic images of malignant cutaneous tumors: (a, b) clinical images of two sebaceous carcinomas located on the scalp of a 63-year-old man affected by the Muir–Torre syndrome. At clinical examination the two lesions appeared as 7 mm flesh-colored papules displaying a central ulceration.
(*Continued*)

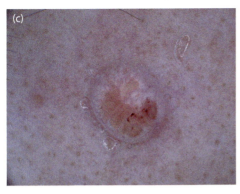 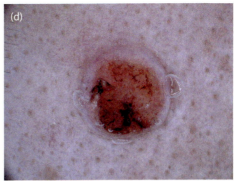

Figure 23.2 (Continued) Clinical and dermoscopic images of benign sebaceous tumors: (c, d) at dermoscopic examination the first lesion had a central ulcerated area surrounded by unfocused linear-irregular vessels; the second lesion was instead characterized by a larger central ulcerated area with polymorphous vessels and some linear unfocused vessels at the periphery.

latter two dermoscopic features are frequently found in several types of cutaneous malignant tumors, both melanocytic and nonmelanocytic.

REFERENCES

1. Shalin SC, Lyle S, Calonje E et al. Sebaceous neoplasia and the Muir-Torre syndrome: Important connections with clinical implications. *Histopathology*. 2010;**56**:133–47.
2. Ollila S, Fitzpatrick R, Sarantaus L et al. The importance of functional testing in the genetic assessment of Muir-Torre syndrome, a clinical subphenotype of HNPCC. *Int J Oncol*. 2006;**28**:149–53.
3. Lallas A, Moscarella E, Argenziano G, Longo C, Apalla Z, Ferrara G, Piana S, Rosato S, Zalaudek I. Dermoscopy of uncommon skin tumours. *Australas J Dermatol*. 2014;**55**(1):53–62.
4. Iacobelli J, Harvey NT, Wood BA. Sebaceous lesions of the skin. *Pathology*. 2017;**49**(7):688–97.
5. John AM, Schwartz RA. Muir-Torre syndrome (MTS): An update and approach to diagnosis and management. *J Am Acad Dermatol*. 2016;**74**(3):558–66.
6. Kim NH, Zell DS, Kolm I et al. The dermoscopic differential diagnosis of yellow lobular-like structures. *Arch Dermatol*. 2008;**144**:962.
7. Moscarella E, Argenziano G, Longo C et al. Clinical, dermoscopic and reflectance confocal microscopy features of sebaceous neoplasms in Muir-Torre syndrome. *J Eur Acad Dermatol Venereol*. 2013;**27**:699–705.
8. Nomura M, Tanaka M, Nunomura M et al. Dermoscopy of rippled pattern sebaceoma. *Dermatol Res Pract*. 2010;**2010**, pii: 140486. Epub 2010 Jul 27.
9. Coates D, Bowling J, Haskett M. Dermoscopic features of extraocular sebaceous carcinoma. *Australas J Dermatol*. 2011;**52**:212–13.

24 Syringocystadenoma papilliferum

Mara Lombardi

INTRODUCTION

Syringocystadenoma papilliferum (SCAP) is a rare, benign hamartomatous adnexal tumor that originates from the apocrine or the eccrine sweat glands.[1] It is a rare neoplasm, presents at birth in 50% of cases or develops during puberty in 15%–30% of cases.[2]

It is frequently seen in association with other benign adnexal lesions, such as apocrine nevus, tubular apocrine adenoma, apocrine hidrocystoma, trichoadenoma, apocrine cystadenoma and clear cell syringoma.[3] SCAP is the most common tumor developing in nevus sebaceous (30% of patients). The most frequent location is the head and neck, with the scalp being the preferential location.[4] Most of the SCAPs are sporadic cases and are diagnosed on histopathology because the clinical presentation is often nonspecific and misleading. Three clinical types have been described: a plaque type presenting as an alopecic patch that may enlarge during puberty to become nodular, verrucous or crusted (often on the scalp); a linear type consisting of multiple reddish-pink firm papules or umbilicated nodules (over face and neck); and a solitary nodular type that are domed pedunculated nodules 5–10 mm in size (often on the trunk) (Figures 24.1 through 24.3).

Histologically it is composed of invaginating cystic spaces open to the skin surface lined by squamous epithelium in the upper portion and sweat gland epithelium in the lower portion.

Histologic examination remains the gold standard in the diagnosis, in addition to complete clinical information.

Local excision when the patient is prepubertal, preferably before enlargement of sebaceous elements, is recommended.

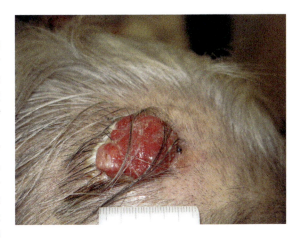

Figure 24.1 Close-up of an exophytic nodular lesion with a lobular surface in the temporal region of the scalp.

Rarely, malignant transformation to basal cell carcinoma (BCC), squamous cell carcinoma (SCC) or sweat gland carcinoma has been documented in plaque and solitary types. Further, SCAP is known to be associated with malignant

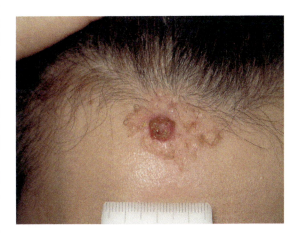

Figure 24.2 Close-up of a verrucous yellowish lesion on the frontal area of the scalp.

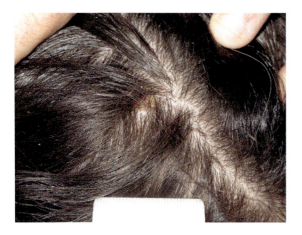

Figure 24.3 Close-up of a plaque in the vertex of the scalp.

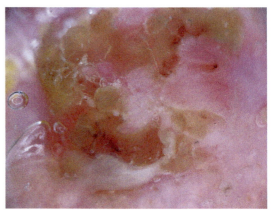

Figure 24.5 Dermatoscopy image of the lesion shows yellow crusts and pinkish-white globular structures with irregular vessels.

tumors, such as BCC, sebaceous carcinoma, verrucous carcinoma and ductal carcinoma. Few cases of malignant transformation of SCAP to syringocystadenocarcinoma papilliferum (SCACP) have been documented until now.[5–7]

DERMOSCOPY

There are few reports in the literature that describe dermoscopic features of syringocystadenoma papilliferum.[8–14] The first description of SCAP associated with nevus sebaceous was reported by Bruno et al.[9]: they described a polymorphous vascular pattern in which some vessels were surrounded by a whitish halo and others were grouped in a horseshoe arrangement on a pinkish-white background.[9] This pattern was also confirmed by Chauhan and colleagues.[14]

Other dermoscopic features observed are a symmetric erythematous lesion with pink-white exophytic papillary structures followed by a central depression, erosions/crust/ulceration and vascular structures (hairpin vessels, polymorphous atypical vessels and common vessels).[7] When it is associated with a nevus sebaceous, a yellow color is also detected (Figures 24.4 through 24.6).[11,13]

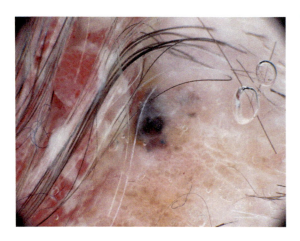

Figure 24.4 Dermatoscopy image of the lesion shows yellow globular-like structures in the background of the lesion and pinkish-white papillary structures together with linear and polymorphous vessels.

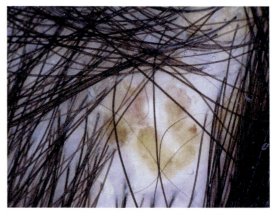

Figure 24.6 Dermatoscopy image of the lesion shows structureless yellow areas with whitish center together with linear vessels.

REFERENCES

1. Yamamoto O, Doi Y, Hamada T et al. An immunohistochemical and ultrastructural study of syringocystoadenoma papilliferum. *Br J Dermatol.* 2002;**147**:936–45.
2. Karg E, Korom I, Varga E et al. Congenital syringocystadenoma papilliferum. *Pediatr Dermatol.* 2008;**25**(1):132–3.
3. Stavrianeas NG, Katoulis AC, Stratigeas NP et al. Development of multiple tumours in a sebaceous nevus of Jadassohn. *Dermatology.* 1997;**195**:155–8.
4. Pahwa P, Kaushal S, Gupta S et al. Linear syringocystadenoma papilliferum: An unusual location. *Pediatr Dermatol.* 2011;**28**(1):61–2.
5. Hoekzema R, Leenarts MF, Nijhuis EW. Syringocystadenocarcinoma papilliferum in a linear nevus verrucosus. *J Cutan Pathol.* 2011;**38**:246–50.
6. Chen J, Beg M, Chen S. Syringocystadenocarcinoma papilliferum *in situ*, a variant of cutaneous adenocarcinoma *in situ*: A case report with literature review. *Am J Dermatopathol.* 2016;**38**:762–5.
7. Satter E, Grady D, Schlocker CT. Syringocystadenocarcinoma papilliferum with locoregional metastases. *Dermatol Online J.* 2014;**20**:22335.
8. Zaballos P, Serrano P, Flores G et al. Dermoscopy of tumours arising in naevus sebaceous: A morphological study of 58 cases. *J Eur Acad Dermatol Venereol.* 2015;**29**:2231–7.
9. Bruno CB, Cordeiro FN, Soares Fdo E et al. Dermoscopic aspects of syringocystadenoma papilliferum associated with nevus sebaceous. *An Bras Dermatol.* 2011;**86**:1213–6.
10. Shindo M, Yamada N, Yoshida Y et al. Syringocystadenoma papilliferum on the male nipple. *J Dermatol.* 2011;**38**:593–6.
11. Duman N, Ersoy-Evans S, Erkin Ozaygen G et al. Syringocystadenoma papilliferum arising on naevus sebaceous: A 6-year-old child case described with dermoscopic features. *Australas J Dermatol.* 2015;**5**:e53–e54.
12. Giorgi V D, Massi D, Trez E et al. Multiple pigmented trichoblastoma and syringocystadenoma papilliferum in naevus sebaceous mimicking a malignant melanoma: A clinical dermoscopic-pathological case study. *Br J Dermatol.* 2003;**149**:1067–70.
13. Lombardi M, Piana S, Longo C et al. Dermoscopy of syringocystadenoma papilliferum. *Australas J Dermatol.* 2018;**59**(1):e59–61.
14. Chauhan P, Chauhan RK, Upadhyaya A et al. Dermoscopy of a rare case of linear syringocystadenoma papilliferum with review of the literature. *Dermatol Pract Concept.* 2018;**8**(1):33–8.

25 Hidradenoma

Riccardo Pampena

INTRODUCTION

Nodular hidradenoma, also called clear cell hidradenoma, eccrine acrospiroma, solid-cystic hidradenoma, clear cell myoepithelioma and eccrine sweat gland adenoma, is an uncommon benign adnexal neoplasm that is currently thought to be of apocrine origin, but in a minority of cases can also be eccrine (poroid hidradenoma).[1] The different variants of hidradenoma cannot be distinguished on a clinical and dermoscopic basis, as in both cases they appear as well-circumscribed, slowly growing nodules with no body site predilection and are more frequently seen in middle-aged patients, with a slight prevalence in females.[2] Histopathologically hidradenoma appears as nonencapsulated solitary

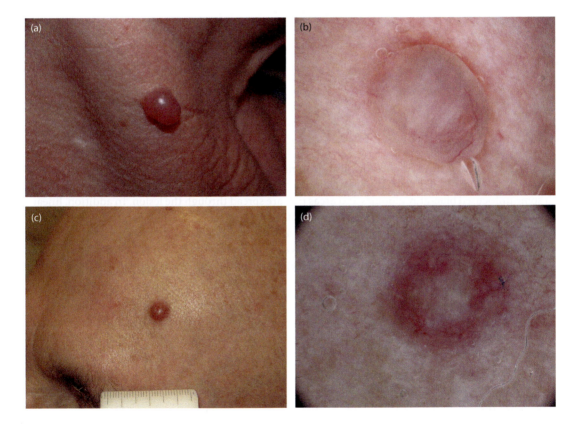

Figure 25.1 Nonpigmented cases of nodular hidradenoma: (a) clinical picture of a 12 mm papule located on the neck of a 70-year-old woman, which appears exophytic and pinkish; (b) dermoscopically, a pinkish background may be seen with diffuse whitish lines and some unfocused linear vessels in the peripheral part of the lesion; (c) clinical image of a 6 mm pinkish papule located on the forehead of a 62-year-old man; (d) at dermoscopic examination a central whitish area may be seen with some whitish lines and roundish structures; at the periphery of the lesion a pinkish area with many unfocused linear-irregular vessels is present.

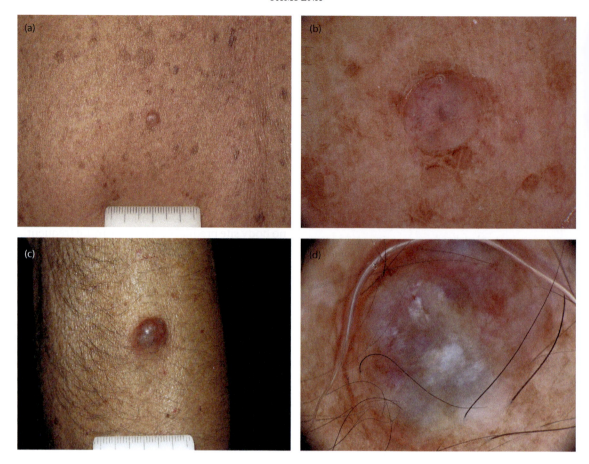

Figure 25.2 Pigmented cases of nodular hidradenoma: (a) clinical picture of a 4 mm flesh-colored papule on the back of a 78-year-old man; (b) pigmentation may only be recognized at dermoscopic examination with some unfocused blue-gray globules and areas that are spread through the lesion. In addition, linear and branching vessels are also present, together with some whitish dots; (c) clinical image of a 10 mm reddish and bluish nodular lesion located on the left arm of a 67-year-old man; (d) dermoscopically, a gray-bluish background may be recognized, with many white streaks mainly located in the central part of the lesion. At the periphery linear-irregular unfocused vessels on a pinkish background may be seen.

dermal nodules that are 1–3 cm in diameter, which may be solid and cystic in different proportions; duct-like structures are also commonly present. Apocrine and eccrine hidradenomas may only be distinguished on histopathologic examination, since the latter are composed of poroid and cuticular cells; while, in the former, clear, polygonal and mucinous cells are present. Clear cells are rich in glycogen and predominate in one-third of cases. The stroma is usually sclerotic.[1] The malignant variant, hidradenocarcinoma, is exceedingly rare and may originate in a preexisting hidradenoma. Because of the very aspecific clinical appearance, the differential diagnosis of hidradenoma includes many other benign and malignant skin tumors, in particular, nonmelanoma skin cancers.[3]

DERMOSCOPY

In 2016 Serrano and colleagues published the largest series of nodular hidradenoma evaluated by dermoscopy.[3] Twenty-eight lesions were considered, of which only one was correctly diagnosed as hidradenoma, while the most common given diagnosis was basal cell carcinoma. The most frequently observed dermoscopic features were pinkish and bluish homogenous areas and white structures, in particular, shiny white lines and amorphous whitish areas. Arborizing and polymorphic (linear, hairpin) vessels were also frequently reported. Interestingly, in all of the considered lesions, other specific criteria for melanocytic and nonmelanocytic lesions were absent. Authors described two different patterns, pigmented and nonpigmented, which were both characterized by whitish structures and vessels, in a bluish background when considering the former and pinkish when considering the latter (Figures 25.1 and 25.2). Other reports also confirmed these findings.[4–7]

REFERENCES

1. Stratigos AJ, Olbricht S, Kwan TH, Bowers KE. Nodular hidradenoma: A report of three cases and review of the literature. *Dermatol Surg*. 1998;**24**:387–91.
2. Zaballos P, Serrano P, Flores G et al. Dermoscopy of tumours arising in naevus sebaceous: A morphological study of 58 cases. *J Eur Acad Dermatol Venereol*. 2015;**29**(11):2231–7.
3. Serrano P, Lallas A, Del Pozo LJ, Karaarslan I, Medina C, Thomas L, Landi C, Argenziano G, Zaballos P. Dermoscopy of nodular hidradenoma, a great masquerader: A morphological study of 28 cases. *Dermatology*. 2016;**232**(1):78–82.
4. Lallas A, Moscarella E, Argenziano G, Longo C, Apalla Z, Ferrara G, Piana S, Rosato S, Zaludek I. Dermoscopy of uncommon skin tumours. *Australas J Dermatol*. 2014;**55**:53–62.
5. Sgambato A, Zalaudek I, Ferrara G, Giorgio CM, Moscarella E, Nicolino R, Argenziano G. Adnexal tumors: Clinical and dermoscopic mimickers of basal cell carcinoma. *Arch Dermatol*. 2008;**144**:426.
6. Yoshida Y, Nakashima K, Yamamoto O. Dermoscopic features of clear cell hidradenoma. *Dermatology*. 2008;**217**:250–1.
7. Robles-Mendez JC, Martínez-Cabriales SA, Villarreal-Martínez A, Ayala-Cortés AS, Miranda Maldonado I, Vázquez-Martínez O, Ocampo-Candiani J. Nodular hidradenoma: Dermoscopic presentation. *J Am Acad Dermatol*. 2017;**76**(2S1):S46–8.

26 Cylindroma and familial cylindromatosis and Brooke–Spiegler syndrome

Riccardo Pampena

INTRODUCTION

Cylindroma is an uncommon benign adnexal tumor probably originating from the secretory coil of the apocrine gland. It usually appears as a solitary skin-colored papular or nodular lesion, located on the head and neck, with a strong predilection for middle-aged and elderly women.[1] Multiple and large variants of cylindromas have been described in the context of two genetic syndromes with autosomal dominant inheritance: familial cylindromatosis (Online Mendelian Inheritance in Man [OMIM] 132700) and Brooke–Spiegler syndrome (OMIM 605041), which represent different phenotypic expressions of mutations in the *CYLD* gene, on chromosome 16q12–q13.[2–4] In the former, which is the rarest condition, only multiple cylindromas may be found, while in Brooke–Spiegler syndrome these are commonly associated with multiple trichoepitheliomas and spiradenomas.[5] In both of these conditions, multiple and coalescing cylindromas may involve the entire scalp, giving a peculiar clinical appearance that has been called "turban tumors."[6] Malignant transformation of cylindroma in cylindrocarcinoma is an exceedingly rare event, which may only occur in long-standing lesions. On histopathologic examination, cylindroma appears as a dermal tumor, which may also involve the subcutis; however, a thin band of uninvolved connective tissue is generally visible between the tumor and the epidermis.

Cylindroma is composed by islands and cords of basaloid cells arranged in a poorly circumscribed mass, characteristically surrounded by a PAS-positive eosinophilic hyaline band. Those cells located at the periphery of tumor islands are smaller and with a basophilic nucleus, while those centrally located are larger and with a vesicular nucleus. A loosely arranged stroma is generally present. Spiradenoma-like areas are sometimes present in cylindromas.[7]

DERMOSCOPY

The dermoscopic appearance of cylindroma has only been described in a limited number of case reports.[8–11] The most reported dermoscopic criteria consisted of arborizing vessels, a white-pinkish background and blue-gray dots/globules (Figure 26.1). On the basis of these findings, cylindroma has been included in the list of adnexal tumors mimicking basal cell carcinoma (BCC). However, arborizing vessels in cylindroma usually differ from those of BCC, mainly because of their blurred appearance, small number of branches and arrangement at the periphery of the lesion (Figure 26.2). In addition, the white-pinkish background is almost never seen in BCC.[12] Furthermore, no specific dermoscopic features have been reported for cylindroma arising in patients with Brooke–Spiegler syndrome or familial cylindromatosis.

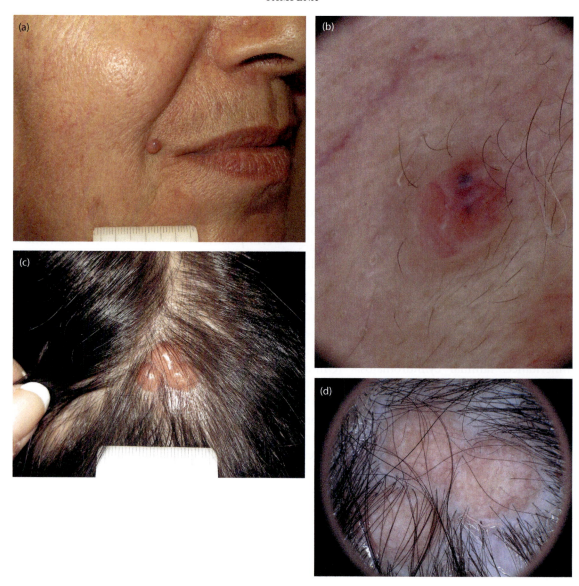

Figure 26.1 Clinical and dermoscopic pictures of two cases of cylindromas: (a) clinical picture of a 5 mm pinkish and bluish papule located at the right labial commissure of a 68-year-old woman; (b) at dermoscopic examination unfocused arborizing vessels and blue-gray areas may be seen on a pinkish background, together with several white lines; (c) clinical image of a 15 mm trilobate flesh-colored mass located on the vertex of a 37-year-old woman; (d) dermoscopically some unfocused linear vessels and white roundish structures may be seen on a pinkish background.

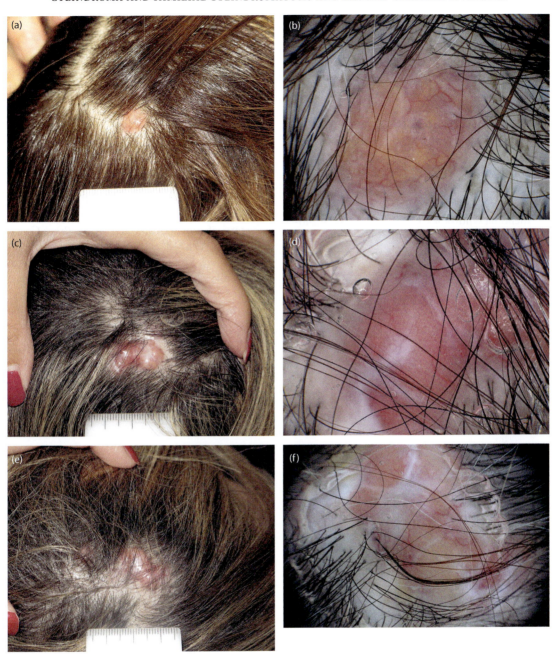

Figure 26.2 Multiple cylindromas located on the scalp of a 52-year-old woman affected by the Brooke–Spiegler syndrome; (a, c, e) at clinical examination multiple pinkish nodules may be seen ranging from 8 to 20 mm; (b, d, f) dermoscopically, the lesions were all characterized by a pinkish background (with a yellow hue in b and f) and unfocused small branched arborizing vessels; white structures (lines in b and septa in d and f) may also be seen.

REFERENCES

1. Rajan N, Ashworth A. Inherited cylindromas: Lessons from a rare tumour. *Lancet Oncol.* 2015;16(9):e460-9.
2. Bowen S, Gill M, Lee DA et al. Mutations in the *CYLD* gene in Brooke-Spiegler syndrome, familial cylindromatosis, and multiple familial trichoepithelioma: Lack of genotype-phenotype correlation. *J Invest Dermatol.* 2005;124:919-20.
3. Young AL, Kellermayer R, Szigeti R et al. *CYLD* mutations underlie Brooke-Spiegler, familial cylindromatosis, and multiple familial trichoepithelioma syndromes. *Clin Genet.* 2006;70:246-9.
4. Saggar S, Chernoff KA, Lodha S et al. *CYLD* mutations in familial skin appendage tumours. *J Med Genet.* 2008;45:298-302.
5. Kazakov DV. Brooke-Spiegler syndrome and phenotypic variants: An update. *Head Neck Pathol.* 2016;10(2):125-30.
6. Jatan A, Cha J, Yeh R, Baldwin M. Modern turban tumour management. *J Plast Reconstr Aesthet Surg.* 2013;66(5):e149-51.
7. Jordão C, de Magalhães TC, Cuzzi T, Ramos-e-Silva M. Cylindroma: An update. *Int J Dermatol.* 2015;54(3):275-8.
8. Lallas A, Apalla Z, Tzellos T et al. Dermoscopy of solitary cylindroma. *Eur J Dermatol.* 2011;21:645-6.
9. Cabo H, Pedrini F, Cohen Sabban E. Dermoscopy of cylindroma. *Dermatol Res Pract.* 2010;2010:pii:285392. Epub 2010 August 24.
10. Jarrett R, Walker L, Bowling J. Dermoscopy of Brooke-Spiegler syndrome. *Arch Dermatol.* 2009;145:854.
11. Cohen YK, Elpern DJ. Dermatoscopic pattern of a cylindroma. *Dermatol Pract Concept.* 2014;4(1):67-8.
12. Lallas A, Moscarella E, Argenziano G, Longo C, Apalla Z, Ferrara G, Piana S, Rosato S, Zalaudek I. Dermoscopy of uncommon skin tumours. *Australas J Dermatol.* 2014;55(1):53-62.

27 Spiradenoma

Riccardo Pampena

INTRODUCTION

Spiradenoma is a benign adnexal tumor originating from apocrine glands. It usually presents as a solitary gray-pinkish nodule, less than 1 cm in diameter, arising on the head and neck or on the truncal region. Moreover, spiradenoma may arise in a sebaceous nevus and is commonly seen in patients affected by the Brooke–Spiegler syndrome. Malignant transformation is rare and has been reported in spiradenomas associated with Brooke–Spiegler syndrome.[1] At histopathologic examination, one or more large dermal nodules are commonly seen, sometimes extending into the subcutis. Within these nodules, two cell populations may be found, consisting of small basaloid cells and more frequent larger cuboidal cells with a pale nucleus. Periodic acid–Schiff (PAS)-positive hyaline material is often present at the periphery of the aggregates, together with a few duct-like structures. In the stroma between lobules, dilatated vessels or even hemorrhage may be seen.[2] Cylindroma-like features are frequently seen in spiradenoma, in particular in patients with Brooke–Spiegler syndrome.

DERMOSCOPY

Only two case reports in the literature described the dermoscopic features of spiradenoma. In one case the presence of a faint grayish-bluish hue and whitish areas was reported (Figure 27.1);[3] in the other case, a structureless pattern and blue clods were described, with the presence of serpentine, branched vessels. Differently from basal cell carcinoma, in which blue clods correspond to pigmented basaloid islands, in spiradenoma this dermoscopic feature seems to correspond to hemorrhage, which is a frequent finding in spiradenoma.[4]

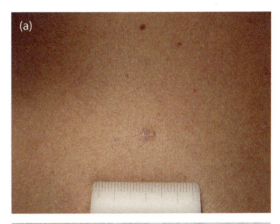

Figure 27.1 Clinical and dermoscopic image of a spiradenoma located on the back of a 30-year-old man: (a) on clinical examination the lesion is composed of a light brown 5 mm macule with a small whitish papule located at the periphery; (b) dermoscopically, a whitish-pinkish background may be seen with a white roundish structure located in the peripheral part.

REFERENCES

1. Kazakov DV. Brooke-Spiegler syndrome and phenotypic variants: An update. *Head Neck Pathol.* 2016;10(2):125–30.
2. Rapini RP. Sweat gland neoplasms. In: Hodgson S, ed. *Practical Dermatopathology*. Philadelphia, PA: Elsevier Mosby; 2005:295.
3. Lallas A, Moscarella E, Argenziano G, Longo C, Apalla Z, Ferrara G, Piana S, Rosato S, Zalaudek I. Dermoscopy of uncommon skin tumours. *Australas J Dermatol.* 2014;55(1):53–62.
4. Tschandl P. Dermatoscopic pattern of a spiradenoma. *Dermatol Pract Concept.* 2012;2(4):204a09.

28 Mammary and extramammary Paget's disease

Riccardo Pampena, Giorgio La Viola, and Alessandro Annetta

INTRODUCTION

Paget's disease usually appears on the breast of adult women with an underlying breast cancer, as a unilateral erythematous/eczematous plaque, which slowly spreads from the nipple to the areola and sometimes to the surrounding skin. In a minority of cases Paget's disease may not be associated with breast cancer, and in 6% of cases it may also involve extramammary sites.[1] Extramammary Paget's disease generally involves body sites with a high density of apocrine glands, primarily the anogenital region, followed by the axillary area. Anecdotic cases have also been reported deriving from modified apocrine glands, such as the ceruminous glands of the external ear and the Moll's glands located on the eyelid. Of note, the mammalian gland is also considered as a modified apocrine gland.[2] The clinical aspect of extramammary Paget's disease is similar to the mammary form; however, crusts or scales are less frequently found because of the location on skin folds; and moreover, it is more frequently seen in elderly men. Rarely both mammary and extramammary Paget's disease may be pigmented.

Concerning the pathogenesis of Paget's disease, the great majority of mammary cases have been associated with direct localization into the basal layer of the epidermis of tumor cells of an underlying intraductal adenocarcinoma of the breast. Regarding extramammary forms, an underlying apocrine carcinoma has been reported in only a quarter of cases; while association with other cancers, such as those of the rectum, prostate, bladder, cervix or urethra, has been reported in 15% of cases. More than half of extramammary cases, together with a minority of mammary forms, are not associated with an underlying malignancy.[1] Generally, Paget's cells are mainly located in the basal layer of the epidermis, but the upper portions may also be involved. These cells are large, pale and characterized by an abundant cytoplasm, rich in mucin (PAS-positive) and pleomorphic nuclei with prominent nucleoli.[3]

DERMOSCOPY

Dermoscopic features of both mammary and extramammary Paget's disease have been described. In nonpigmented forms, milky-red areas, irregular linear vessels and shiny white lines were the most reported criteria. Moreover, in mammary forms, surface scales were often visible at clinical and dermoscopic examination, differently from extramammary forms (Figures 28.1 and 28.2).[4,5] In pigmented cases, the presence of a light brown diffuse pigmentation and peppering-like blue-gray dots may be seen, in various combinations with the previously reported nonpigmented criteria.[6,7] Because of the presence of regression-like features, such as white areas and peppering-like blue-gray dots, differential diagnosis with melanoma should always be considered.[7,8] Other differential diagnoses include Bowen disease, basal cell carcinoma, eczematous dermatitis, psoriasis, fungal infection and erosive adenomatosis of the nipple.[1,2,9] When considering the differential diagnosis of extramammary Paget's disease with eczematous dermatitis and fungal infections, it was seen that the former more frequently displayed milky-red areas and vascular structures.[4]

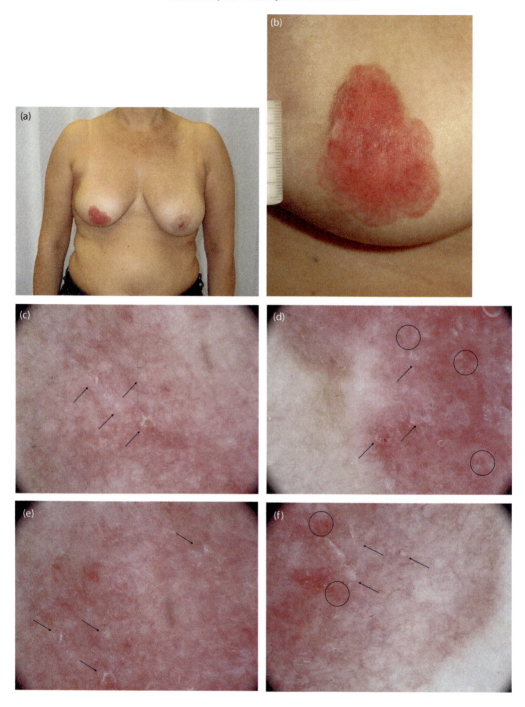

Figure 28.1 Clinical and dermoscopic images of a case of mammary Paget's disease: (a, b) clinical pictures of a 5 cm erythematous plaque involving the right breast of a 50-year-old woman affected by an underlying intraductal adenocarcinoma of the breast. The plaque involved the nipple, the areola and the surrounding skin of the breast. Erythema appeared more intense in the central part and progressively faded moving toward the periphery. (c–f) At dermoscopic examination milky-red areas (black circles), irregular linear vessels (f) and scales (black arrows) may be seen.

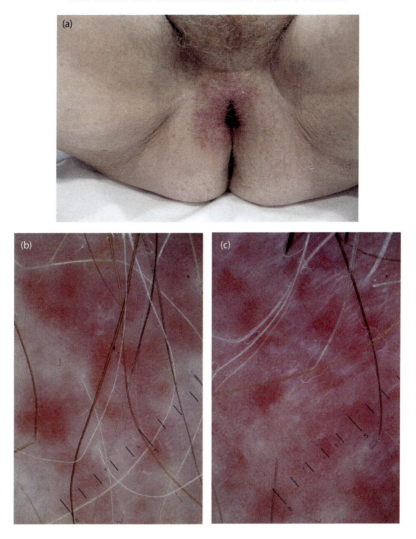

Figure 28.2 Clinical and dermoscopic images of a case of extramammary Paget's disease: (a) on clinical examination an erythematous perianal macule with some peripheral isolated small lesions may be seen in a 77-year-old woman; (b, c) dermoscopically diffuse dotted vessels are visible on a pinkish-reddish background with whitish streaks.

REFERENCES

1. Lloyd J, Flanagan AM. Mammary and extramammary Paget's disease. *J Clin Pathol*. 2000;**53**:742–9.
2. Wagner G, Sachse MM. Extramammary Paget disease – Clinical appearance, pathogenesis, management. *J Dtsch Dermatol Ges*. 2011;**9**:448–54.
3. Sandoval-Leon AC, Drews-Elger K, Gomez-Fernandez CR, Yepes MM, Lippman ME. Paget's disease of the nipple. *Breast Cancer Res Treat*. 2013;**141**(1):1–12.
4. Mun JH, Park SM, Kim GW, Song M, Kim HS, Ko HC, Kim BS, Kim MB. Clinical and dermoscopic characteristics of extramammary Paget disease: A study of 35 cases. *Br J Dermatol*. 2016;**174**(5):1104–7.
5. Crignis GS, Abreu Ld, Buçard AM, Barcaui CB. Polarized dermoscopy of mammary Paget disease. *An Bras Dermatol*. 2013;**88**(2):290–2.
6. Longo C, Fantini F, Cesinaro AM, Bassoli S, Seidenari S, Pellacani G. Pigmented mammary Paget disease: Dermoscopic, *in vivo* reflectance-mode confocal microscopic, and

immunohistochemical study of a case. *Arch Dermatol.* 2007;**143**(6):752–4.
7. Coras-Stepanek B, von Portatius A, Dyall-Smith D, Stolz W. Dermatoscopy of pigmented extramammary Paget disease simulating melanoma. *J Am Acad Dermatol.* 2012;**67**(4):e144–6.
8. Yanagishita T, Tamada Y, Tanaka M, Kasugai C, Takahashi E, Matsumoto Y, Watanabe D. Pigmented mammary Paget disease mimicking melanoma on dermatoscopy. *J Am Acad Dermatol.* 2011;**64**(6):e114–6.
9. Errichetti E, Avellini C, Pegolo E, De Francesco V. Dermoscopy as a supportive instrument in the early recognition of erosive adenomatosis of the nipple and mammary Paget's disease. *Ann Dermatol.* 2017;**29**(3):365–7.

29 Syringoma

Riccardo Pampena

INTRODUCTION

Syringoma is a benign adnexal tumor deriving from intraepidermal eccrine ducts, which is usually found as multiple papules, ranging from 1 to 3 mm in diameter, on the lower eyelids and cheeks of young females.[1] The papules are skin-colored or yellowish and generally asymptomatic. Solitary, giant, plaque-like, milia-like, linear unilateral and eruptive forms have also been reported, as well as location in other body areas, such as the genital area, skin folds and scalp.[2-6] The clinical aspect of these uncommon variants has been reported to be similar to the classic form. Histopathologically, syringoma appears as a dermal tumor composed of a dense fibrous stroma in which multiple small ducts

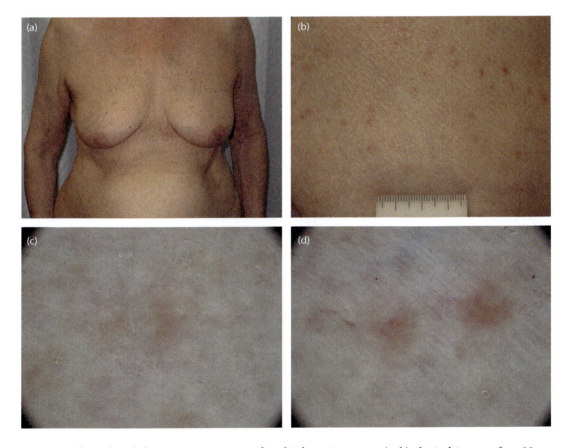

Figure 29.1 Clinical and dermoscopic images of multiple syringomas: (a, b) clinical image of an 80-year-old woman with multiple syringomas located on her breast area with a bilateral distribution. On clinical examination lesions appeared as small (1–2 mm in diameter) erythematous papules; (c, d) dermoscopically a yellowish-brownish background may be seen with some fine linear vessels.

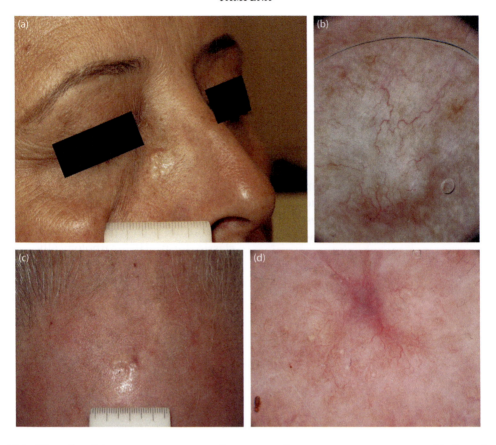

Figure 29.2 Clinical and dermoscopic pictures of two cases of syringomatous carcinoma: (a) clinical picture of a plaque scar-like whitish lesion located on the nose of a 56-year-old woman; (b) at dermoscopic examination a whitish background may be seen with many linear and branching vessels and some pigmented brownish areas; (c) clinical image of a plaque scar-like flesh-colored lesion, centrally depressed, located on the scalp of a 65-year-old man; (d) dermoscopically, several linear and arborizing vessels may be found on a whitish-pinkish background; some milia-like cysts were also visible.

lined by two layers of cuboidal cells may be recognized; keratinous cysts may also be seen. In the clear cell variant of syringoma, the epithelial cells lining the ducts contain abundant glycogen and appear larger and paler. This variant is frequently associated with diabetes mellitus.[7] The malignant form of syringoma is called syringomatous carcinoma, which is thought not to derive from the malignant degeneration of syringoma, but to originate as a malignant tumor *ab initio*. The differential diagnosis of syringoma is very wide and mainly related to body site and lesion number. Milia represent the most important differential diagnosis of the classic variant.[1]

DERMOSCOPY

The dermoscopic appearance of syringoma was first described in 2011 by Hayashi et al., who reported a case of unilateral linear syringoma. Dermoscopic examination revealed multifocal whitish structures on a homogenous brown background and a delicate peripheral pigmented network.[8] Lallas et al. in 2014 reported a case of eruptive syringomas, which was characterized by fine linear vessels on a yellowish-brownish background (Figure 29.1).[9] Subsequently, two other authors described the dermoscopic findings of eruptive syringomas, reporting the common finding of a fine pigmented network and a reddish tinge or rosettes.[3,10] In 2017, Corazza and colleagues described the dermoscopic appearance of an isolated syringoma located on the vulva. They observed a pinkish background with multiple yellow-whitish roundish structures; dotted and linear vessels were also seen.[2] Dermoscopic features of syringomatous carcinoma were also reported in the literature; in particular, fine linear-branched vessels with a white to pink homogenous background and surface scales were observed (Figure 29.2).[11]

REFERENCES

1. Williams K, Shinkai K. Evaluation and management of the patient with multiple syringomas: A systematic review of the literature. *J Am Acad Dermatol.* 2016;**74**:1234–40.e9.
2. Corazza M, Borghi A, Minghetti S, Ferron P, Virgili A. Dermoscopy of isolated syringoma of the vulva. *J Am Acad Dermatol.* 2017;**76**(2S1):S37–9.
3. Sakiyama M, Maeda M, Fujimoto N, Satoh T. Eruptive syringoma localized in intertriginous areas. *J Dtsch Dermatol Ges.* 2014;**12**:72–3.
4. Kirshbaum B, Rosenberg PE. Syringoma. *Arch Dermatol.* 1969;**100**:372–3.
5. Kikuchi I, Idemori M, Okazaki M. Plaque type syringoma. *J Dermatol.* 1979;**6**:329–31.
6. Weiss E, Paez E, Greenberg AS, San Juan E, Fundaminsky M, Helfman TA. Eruptive syringomas associated with milia. *Int J Dermatol.* 1995;**34**:193–5.
7. Danialan R, Mutyambizi K, Aung P, Prieto VG, Ivan D. Challenges in the diagnosis of cutaneous adnexal tumours. *J Clin Pathol.* 2015;**68**(12):992–1002.
8. Hayashi Y, Tanaka M, Nakajima S, Ozeki M, Inoue T, Ishizaki S, Fujibayashi M. Unilateral linear syringoma in a Japanese female: Dermoscopic differentiation from lichen planus linearis. *Dermatol Reports.* 2011;**3**(3):e42.
9. Lallas A, Moscarella E, Argenziano G, Longo C, Apalla Z, Ferrara G, Piana S, Rosato S, Zalaudek I. Dermoscopy of uncommon skin tumours. *Australas J Dermatol.* 2014;**55**(1):53–62.
10. Zhong P, Tan C. Dermoscopic features of eruptive milium-like syringoma. *Eur J Dermatol.* 2015;**25**(2):203–4.
11. Nojima K, Namiki T, Hanafusa T, Miura K, Yokozeki H. Syringomatous carcinoma and its dermoscopic features. *Australas J Dermatol.* 2017;**58**(3):e152–3.

30 Eccrine poroma and eccrine porocarcinoma

Riccardo Pampena

INTRODUCTION

Eccrine poroma is a benign adnexal tumor derived from the acrosyringium of sweat glands, generally arising in middle-aged or elderly patients. It may appear in any body sites with sweat glands and simulate many other benign and malignant cutaneous lesions. It is classically defined as a solitary nodule located on acral sites and surrounded by a collarette scale.[1] Histopathologically it consists of cords and columns of small and PAS-positive basaloid cells extending from the basis of the epidermis into the dermis; sometimes ductal structures are also present. Eccrine poroma belongs to a spectrum of eccrine benign tumors originating from the ductal cells of sweat glands, which also comprises the dermal duct tumor and the hidroacanthoma simplex. In the former, islands of basaloid cells resembling those of eccrine poroma are located deeper in the dermis; in the latter these are instead located within the epidermis. In addition, a minority of poromas have an apocrine origin and are commonly located on the head and neck region.[2] Porocarcinoma represents the malignant variant of eccrine poroma, which may originate *de novo* or in the context of a long-standing and untreated eccrine poroma. The risk of malignant transformation indicates surgical excision as the best approach in the management of eccrine poroma.[3] On histopathology porocarcinoma is composed of intraepidermal islands and nests of atypical small basaloid cells and cords and columns of large atypical cells extending into the dermis.[2]

DERMOSCOPY

A high degree of variability has been reported for poroma concerning its dermoscopic

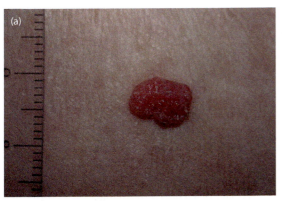 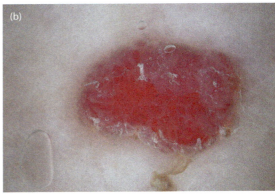

Figure 30.1 Clinical and dermoscopic images of a case of eccrine poroma located on the back of a 73-year-old man: (a) on clinical examination the lesion appears as a nonpigmented 7 mm papule with a central ulcerated area; (b) dermoscopically, some linear vessels, milky-red globules and white interlacing areas around vessels may be seen.

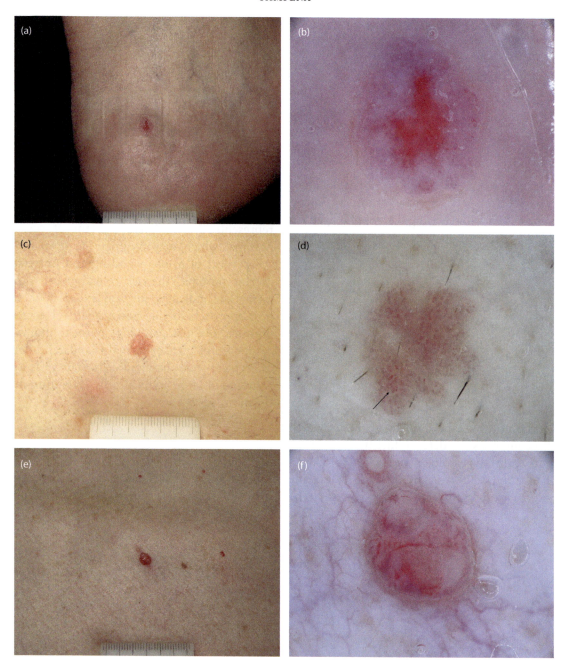

Figure 30.2 Clinical and dermoscopic features of four cases of eccrine poroma: (a) clinical picture of a 6 mm flesh-colored papular lesion, located on the heel of a 70-year-old man. A central ulceration may be seen; (b) dermoscopic examination displayed a collarette, milky-red globules in the central ulcerated area and some dotted vessels in the peripheral part of the lesion; (c) clinical image of a 8 mm pinkish macular lesion located on the pectoral area of a 69-year-old man; (d) dermoscopically, polymorphous vessels are visible with white interlacing areas around the vessels. Some branching vessels with rounded endings, also called "chalice-form" or "cherry-blossoms" vessels, may be seen in the lower part of the lesion (black arrow); (e) clinical image of a 5 mm reddish papule located on the pectoral area of a 42-year-old man; (f) dermoscopically, linear and branched vessels are visible on a pinkish background. *(Continued)*

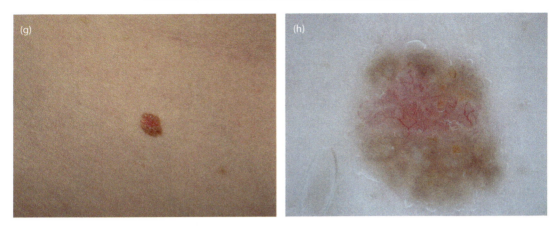

Figure 30.2 (Continued) Clinical and dermoscopic features of four cases of eccrine poroma: (g) clinical image of a 10 mm plaque with a reddish center and peripheral pigmentation located on the abdomen of a 39-year-old woman; (h) on dermoscopy, in the central reddish area many arborizing vessels may be seen; however, at the periphery, some yellowish scales and whitish, roundish structures are visible, over a brownish background.

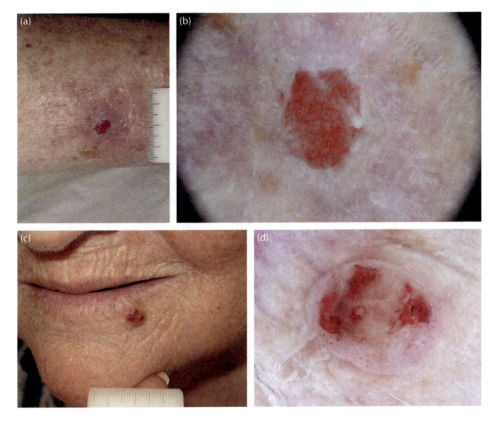

Figure 30.3 Clinical and dermoscopic images of two cases of porocarcinoma: (a) clinical image of a 10 mm ulcerated papule on the leg of a 92-year-old woman; (b) on dermoscopic examination a central ulcerated area may be seen with polymorphous vessels; whitish structures are instead present at the periphery of the lesion; (c) clinical pictures of a 7 mm pinkish and partially ulcerated papule, located below the left side of the lower lip of a 75-year-old woman; (d) at dermoscopic examination some ulcerated areas are visible, together with polymorphic vessels (dotted and linear irregular vessels) on a pinkish background.

appearance, which may be explained by the existence of different histopathologic subtypes.[4] Pigmented forms of poroma have also been described.[5]

Many different dermoscopic criteria have been reported in poromas, such as a polymorphous vascular pattern, perivascular whitish halo, arborizing vessels and blue-gray globules/nests, which may explain why this tumor may frequently simulate other cutaneous lesions, in particular, basal cell carcinoma, but also squamous cells carcinoma, seborrheic keratosis and amelanotic melanoma. However, a wider list of clinical and dermoscopic differential diagnoses has been reported for this chameleonic tumor.[1]

The dermoscopic features associated with poroma have been mainly reported in small case series;[6–13] however, in 2017 Marchetti et al.[1] performed a blinded study using control lesions to assess dermoscopic criteria independently associated with poroma diagnoses, which are white interlacing areas around vessels, yellow structureless areas, milky-red globules and vessels poorly visualized (Figure 30.1).

They also defined four clinical/dermoscopic patterns for poroma, even though some lesions did not fit with any of these groups. The first was most commonly seen on hands and feet and frequently displayed a collarette, blood spots, yellow structureless areas, milky-red globules, milky-red areas and branched vessels with rounded endings. The latter dermoscopic features were also described as "chalice-form" and "cherry-blossoms" vessels (Figure 30.2a, b).[14]

The second was found on the trunk and extremities but not on acral regions and was frequently characterized by polymorphous vessels, white interlacing areas around vessels and branched vessels with rounded endings (Figure 30.2c, d). The third was mainly found in small lesions with no body site predilection; vessels were often absent or characterized by branched vessels with rounded endings (Figure 30.2e, f).

The fourth pattern was instead characteristic of large lesions, without any body predilection, and was also reported in pigmented poromas; on dermoscopic examination blood spots were frequently found, as well as keratin/scale and atypical hairpin vessels[1] (Figure 30.2g, h).

Concerning porocarcinoma, a polymorphous vascular pattern (dotted, linear irregular vessels) and ulceration were the most commonly reported dermoscopic criteria (Figure 30.3).[15–20]

REFERENCES

1. Marchetti MA, Marino ML, Virmani P et al. Dermoscopic features and patterns of poromas: A multicentre observational case-control study conducted by the International Dermoscopy Society. *J Eur Acad Dermatol Venereol*. 2017 December 1. [Epub ahead of print].
2. Sawaya JL, Khachemoune A. Poroma: A review of eccrine, apocrine, and malignant forms. *Int J Dermatol*. 2014;**53**(9):1053–61.
3. Sgouros D, Piana S, Argenziano G, Longo C, Moscarella E, Karaarslan IK, Akalin T, Ozdemir F, Zalaudek I. Clinical, dermoscopic and histopathological features of eccrine poroid neoplasms. *Dermatology*. 2013;**227**(2):175–9.
4. Lallas A, Chellini PR, Guimarães MG, Cordeiro N, Apalla Z, Longo C, Moscarella E, Alfano R, Argenziano G. Eccrine poroma: The great dermoscopic imitator. *J Eur Acad Dermatol Venereol*. 2016;**30**(10):e61–3.
5. Bombonato C, Piana S, Moscarella E, Lallas A, Argenziano G, Longo C. Pigmented eccrine poroma: Dermoscopic and confocal features. *Dermatol Pract Concept*. 2016;**6**(3):59–62.
6. Shalom A, Schein O, Landi C et al. Dermoscopic findings in biopsy-proven poromas. *Dermatol Surg*. 2012;**38**:1091–6.
7. Avilés-Izquierdo JA, Velázquez-Tarjuelo D, Lecona-Echevarría M et al. Dermoscopic features of eccrine poroma. *Actas Dermosifiliogr*. 2009;**100**:133–6.
8. Nicolino R, Zalaudek I, Ferrara G et al. Dermoscopy of eccrine poroma. *Dermatology*. 2007;**215**:160–3.
9. Nishikawa Y, Kaneko T, Takiyoshi N et al. Dermoscopy of eccrine poroma with calcification. *J Dermatol Case Rep*. 2009;**3**:38–40.
10. Ferrari A, Buccini P, Silipo V et al. Eccrine poroma: A clinical dermoscopic study of seven cases. *Acta Derm Venereol*. 2009;**89**:160–4.

11. Kuo H-W, Ohara K. Pigmented eccrine poroma: A report of two cases and study with dermatoscopy. *Dermatol Surg.* 2003;**29**:1076–9.
12. Altamura D, Piccolo D, Lozzi GP et al. Eccrine poroma in an unusual site: A clinical and dermoscopic simulator of amelanotic melanoma. *J Am Acad Dermatol.* 2005;**53**:539–41.
13. Brugués A, Gamboa M, Alós L, Carrera C, Malvehy J, Puig S. The challenging diagnosis of eccrine poromas. *J Am Acad Dermatol.* 2016;**74**(6):e113–5.
14. Espinosa AE, Ortega BC, Venegas RQ, Ramírez RG. Dermoscopy of non-pigmented eccrine poromas: Study of Mexican cases. *Dermatol Pract Concept.* 2013;**3**(1):25–8.
15. Suzaki R, Shioda T, Konohana I, Ishizaki S, Sawada M, Tanaka M. Dermoscopic features of eccrine porocarcinoma arising from hidroacanthoma simplex. *Dermatol Res Pract.* 2010;**2010**:192371.
16. Edamitsu T, Minagawa A, Koga H, Uhara H, Okuyama R. Eccrine porocarcinoma shares dermoscopic characteristics with eccrine poroma: A report of three cases and review of the published work. *J Dermatol.* 2016;**43**(3):332–5.
17. Godinez-Puig V, Martini MC, Yazdan P, Yoo SS. Dermoscopic findings in porocarcinoma. *Dermatol Surg.* 2017;**43**(5):744–5.
18. Pinheiro R, Oliveira A, Mendes-Bastos P. Dermoscopic and reflectance confocal microscopic presentation of relapsing eccrine porocarcinoma. *J Am Acad Dermatol.* 2017;**76**(2S1):S73–5.
19. Dong H, Zhang H, Liu N, Soyer HP. Dermoscopy of a pigmented apocrine porocarcinoma arising from a pigmented hidroacanthoma simplex. *Australas J Dermatol.* 2018;**59**(2):e151–2.
20. Blum A, Metzler G, Bauer J. Polymorphous vascular patterns in dermoscopy as a sign of malignant skin tumors. A case of an amelanotic melanoma and a porocarcinoma. *Dermatology.* 2005;**210**(1):58–9.

SECTION IV

Mesenchymal Tumors

31 Dermatofibrosarcoma protuberans
Elisa Benati

INTRODUCTION

Dermatofibrosarcoma protuberans (DFSP), also known as dermatofibrosarcoma of Darier and Ferrand, is a rare fibrohistiocytic tumor of intermediate- to low-grade malignancy. Taylor first described it in 1890, but Darier was credited with establishing DFSP as a distinct clinicopathologic entity in 1924, and finally, Hoffman established the term in 1925. Overall annual incidence has been estimated to be 4.2 per million, and the tumor accounts for approximately 0.1% of all malignancies. The incidence is almost double among blacks compared to whites, and women have a higher incidence rate than men; the highest age-specific annual incidence rates are observed between the ages of 30 and 50 years. Most occur on the trunk, followed by the upper extremities, lower extremities, and head and neck. Infrequently, it may affect the genitalia. DFSP in children has been reported to represent around 8% of cases, 15% of them being congenital. The distribution is similar to that in adults.

Approximately 10% of DFSP report prior trauma, surgical or burn scars, and even immunizations at the site of disease, but a causative relationship is unclear. Because of its rarity, slow progression and lack of early clinical clues, the diagnosis of DFSP is often delayed. Classical DFSP clinically appeared like indurated, irregularly shaped plaques exhibiting flesh to reddish-brown color (Figure 31.1a, b). Some lesions also showed thin telangiectasia on the surface. Less frequently, a morphea-like, angioma-like, atrophic, violaceous plaque without nodularity is found. Angioma-like DFSP presented as small, red and hard-elastic papules with smooth surface and superficial telangiectasia; a keloid-like variant showed up as a pink-to-red firm translucent mass with smooth surface and telangiectasia; a morphea-like variant clinically appeared as a white-to-brown atrophic plaque with irregularly shaped edges; and a nodular morphea-like variant appeared as a hardened, livid nodule with smooth surface surrounded by a whitish morphea-like plaque. DFSP

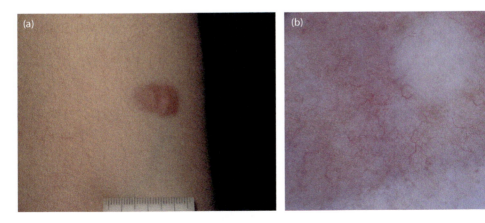

Figure 31.1 Clinical image of a DFSP: (a) an indurated, irregularly shaped plaque. (b) Dermoscopy revealed a structureless depigmented area and irregular branched vessels on a red pale background.

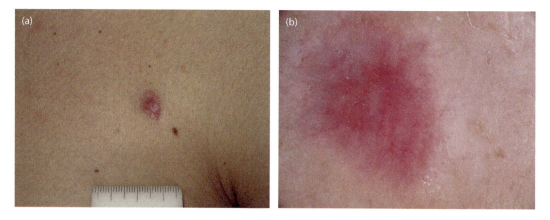

Figure 31.2 (a) Clinical view reveals a red nodule. (b) Dermoscopy image shows the presence of branched vessels, pink background and structureless hypopigmented areas.

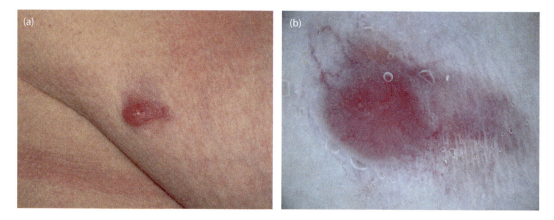

Figure 31.3 (a) Clinical view reveals a red nodule on the breast. This is an angioma-like variant. (b) Dermoscopy image shows the presence of linear irregular and branched vessels arranging in a centrifugal fashion on a pinkish background.

on black skin presented as a very large, partially pigmented, infiltrated plaque, whose surface was surmounted by pinkish to red nodules. Clinical differential diagnosis includes neurofibroma, leiomyoma, malignant melanoma, morpheaform basal cell carcinoma, keloid, desmoid tumors, Kaposi's sarcoma, fibrosarcoma, dermatofibroma, nodular fasciitis and sarcoidosis.

DERMOSCOPY

DFSP under dermoscopy is characterized by multicomponent patterns; the following structures were the most detected: delicate pigmented network, branched vessels, structureless light brown areas, white streaks, pink background and structureless hypo- or depigmented areas (Figure 31.2a, b). When visible, vessels mostly showed an arborizing pattern. Rare variants include an angioma-like variant that shows thick, arborizing vessels arranging in a centrifugal fashion on a pinkish background (Figure 31.3a, b); a keloid-like variant that is characterized by polymorphic vessels (either linear or arborizing) on a white-to-bluish background, and structureless white areas were also detectable; a morphea-like variant that reveals in the inner portion hypopigmented structures, surrounded by a slightly pigmented network with linear vessels; and a nodular morphea-like variant that is shown at dermoscopic examination—the peripheral plaque showed a slightly pigmented network, arborizing thin vessels and hypopigmented unstructured areas on a pinkish background, whereas the inner nodular portion exhibited a dotted vascular pattern and white streaks. Dermoscopic examination of DFSP on black skin showed an atypical network, shiny white streaks, unfocused linear-irregular vessels and hyper- or hypopigmented areas.[1-4]

REFERENCES

1. Costa C, Cappello M, Argenziano G, Piccolo V, Scalvenzi M. Dermoscopy of uncommon variants of dermatofibrosarcoma protuberans. *JEADV*. 2017;**31**:e349–85.
2. Deinlein T, Richtig G, Schwab C, Scarfi F, Arzberger E, Wolf I, Hofmann-Wellenhof R, Zalaudek I. The use of dermatoscopy in diagnosis and therapy of nonmelanocytic skin cancer. *J Dtsch Dermatol Ges*. 2016;**14**(2):144–51.
3. Acosta AE, Velez CS. Dermatofibrosarcoma protuberans. *Curr Treat Options Oncol*. 2017;**18**(9):56.
4. Bernard J, Poulalhon N, Argenziano G, Debarbieux S, Dalle S, Thomas L. Dermoscopy of dermatofibrosarcoma protuberans: A study of 15 cases. *Br J Dermatol*. 2013;**169**(1):85–90.

32 Atypical fibroxanthoma

Elisa Benati

INTRODUCTION

Atypical fibroxanthoma (AFX) is a rare, low-grade superficial sarcoma of fibrous tissue, a spindle cell neoplasm. It is considered a superficial variant of undifferentiated pleomorphic sarcoma (formerly known as malignant fibrous histiocytoma). Although atypical fibroxanthoma has similar histologic features to undifferentiated pleomorphic sarcoma, it behaves less aggressively. It has locally aggressive behavior and a tendency to recur after surgery. However, its metastatic potential is low. It is most often found on the head and neck on sun-damaged skin in elderly patients. Clinically, it manifests as a rapidly enlarging, reddish, dome-shaped nodule, often with an eroded or crusted surface (Figures 32.1a, b and 32.2a, b). Less often the tumor acquires a darker hue due to hemosiderin deposition. AFX can be added to the list of slightly pigmented, reddish, malignant cutaneous tumors, such as squamous cell carcinoma, Merkel cell carcinoma, amelanotic/hypomelanotic melanoma and eccrine porocarcinoma, displaying prominent and chaotic dermatoscopic neoangiogenetic features in more advanced stages of proliferation. The "EFG rule," which recommends excision of any skin lesion with the clinical features of *e*levation, *f*irmness and *g*rowth, ensured this kind of lesion was removed and subjected to histopathologic examination.

DERMOSCOPY

Dermoscopically, AFX displays reddish and whitish areas in combination with a polymorphous vascular pattern comprising dotted, short, fine linear and thick irregular linear vessels; moreover, ulceration and hemorrhage can be present (Figures 32.3 through 32.5). Like Merkel cell carcinoma, although findings of AFX cannot be regarded as specific, dermoscopy minimizes the risk of evaluating the tumor as benign. Specifically, detection of

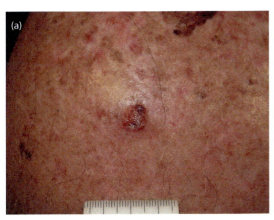 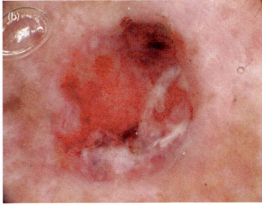

Figure 32.1 (a) Clinical image of an atypical fibroxanthoma arising on the scalp of a 73-year-old man. (b) Dermoscopy reveals reddish and whitish areas in combination with polymorphous vessels and ulceration.

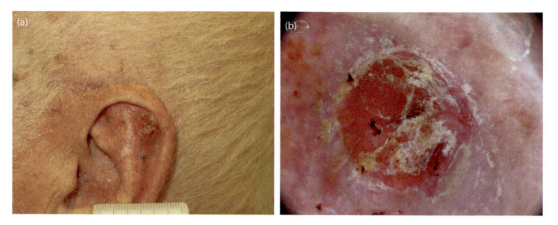

Figure 32.2 (a) Clinical image reveals a red nodule with scales of the ear in a 79-year-old man. (b) Dermoscopy reveals reddish area in combination with ulceration, crusts and scales.

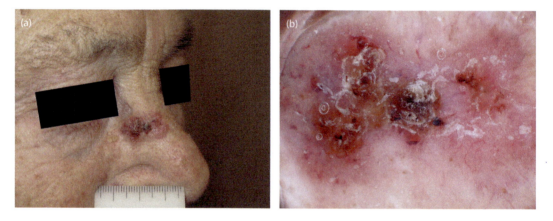

Figure 32.3 (a) Clinical view reveals a red plaque on the nose in an elderly patient. (b) Dermoscopy image shows the presence of a reddish area with a polymorphous vascular pattern comprising dotted and short irregular linear vessels; moreover, ulceration and crusts are present.

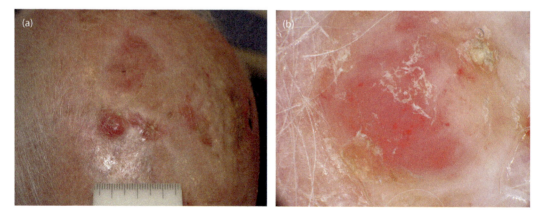

Figure 32.4 (a) Clinical view reveals a red nodule on a photo-damaged scalp. (b) Dermoscopy image shows the presence of dotted and linear irregular vessels and milky-red areas.

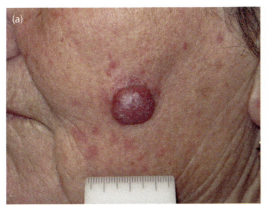
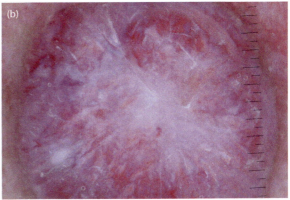

Figure 32.5 (a) A case of atypical fibroxanthoma characterized by a red nodule of a cheek. (b) Dermoscopy image shows the presence of polymorphous not focused vessels and whitish area.

a polymorphous vascular pattern should raise suspicion of a malignant tumor, warranting complete surgical excision. A delicate pigment network has also been described in DFSP, but it lacks the characteristic peripheral arrangement observed in dermatofibroma.[1-5]

REFERENCES

1. Bugatti L, Filosa G. Dermatoscopic features of cutaneous atypical fibroxanthoma: Three cases. *Clin Exp Dermatol.* 2009;**34**(8):e898–900.
2. Inskip M, Magee J, Weedon D, Rosendahl C. Atypical fibroxanthoma of the cheek—Case report with dermatoscopy and dermatopathology. *Dermatol Pract Concept.* 2014;**4**(2):77–80.
3. Soleymani T, Tyler Hollmig S. Conception and management of a poorly understood spectrum of dermatologic neoplasms: Atypical fibroxanthoma, pleomorphic dermal sarcoma, and undifferentiated pleomorphic sarcoma. *Curr Treat Options Oncol.* 2017;**18**(8):50.
4. Lallas A, Moscarella E, Argenziano G, Longo C, Apalla Z, Ferrara G, Piana S, Rosato S, Zalaudek I. Dermoscopy of uncommon skin tumours. *Australas J Dermatol.* 2014;**55**(1):53–62.
5. Moscarella E, Piana S, Specchio F et al. Dermoscopy features of atypical fibroxanthoma: A multicenter study of the International Dermoscopy Society. *Australas J Dermatol.* 2018;**59**(4):309–14.

33 Malignant fibrous histiocytoma (pleomorphic undifferentiated sarcoma)

Elisa Benati

INTRODUCTION

Malignant fibrous histiocytoma (MFH) was first described in 1961 by Kauffman and Stout[1]; MFH is the most common soft tissue sarcoma in late adulthood. It is much more aggressive than atypical fibroxanthoma, with higher recurrence and higher metastatic rates. MFH typically appears between the sixth and eighth decade of life, although childhood tumors have been reported. It has a slight male predominance (nearly 3:1). The head and neck are the most common locations followed closely by the extremities; tumors on upper extremities occur almost twice as often as those on the thighs or legs. Similar to AFX, cutaneous undifferentiated pleomorphic sarcomas are predominantly found on actinically damaged skin in elderly individuals. There is no clinically characteristic presentation that allows for differentiation from other sarcomas. They usually present as solitary, firm nodules with a brownish to erythematous color. Here, too, squamous cell carcinoma, basal cell carcinoma, amelanotic melanoma and other kinds of sarcoma have to be considered in the differential diagnosis.

DERMOSCOPY

Dermoscopically, MFH displays shiny white-red structureless areas in combination with a polymorphous vascular pattern (Figure 33.1a, b). White streaks and rosettes can also be observed. The dermoscopic findings cannot be regarded as specific; as in AFX, dermoscopy minimizes the risk of evaluating the tumor as benign. Specifically, detection of a polymorphous vascular pattern should raise suspicion of a malignant tumor, warranting complete surgical excision.[1-5]

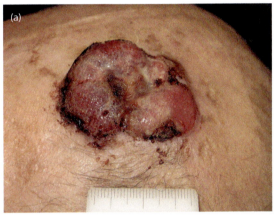

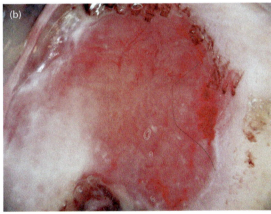

Figure 33.1 (a) Clinical view reveals an ulcerated nodule on the scalp of an 82-year-old man. (b) Dermoscopy image shows the presence of a reddish and whitish area with a polymorphous vascular pattern comprising dotted and irregular linear vessels; moreover, ulceration and crusts are present.

REFERENCES

1. Love WE, Schmitt AR, Bordeaux JS. Management of unusual cutaneous malignancies: Atypical fibroxanthoma, malignant fibrous histiocytoma, sebaceous carcinoma, extramammary Paget disease. *Dermatol Clin.* 2011;29(2):201–16, viii.
2. Salerni G, Alonso C, Sanchez-Granel G, Gorosito M. Dermoscopic findings in an early malignant fibrous histiocytoma on the face. *Dermatol Pract Concept.* 2017;7(3):44–6.
3. Kohlmeyer J, Steimle-Grauer SA, Hein R. Cutaneous sarcomas. *J Dtsch Dermatol Ges.* 2017;15(6):630–48.
4. Mentzel T. Sarcomas of the skin in the elderly. *Clin Dermatol.* 2011;29(1):80–90.
5. Suzuki S, Watanabe S, Kato H, Inagaki H, Hattori H, Morita A. A case of cutaneous malignant fibrous histiocytoma with multiple organ metastases. *Kaohsiung J Med Sci.* 2013;29(2):111–5.

SECTION V

Other Uncommon Tumors

34 Merkel cell carcinoma

Elisa Benati

INTRODUCTION

Merkel cell carcinoma (MCC) is a rare, very aggressive neuroendocrine tumor of the skin characterized by frequent recurrences and early metastatic spread. The incidence of MCC has tripled in recent years and is today estimated at about 0.24 per 100,000 person-years. MCC shows a predilection for elderly white men and immunosuppressed patients. Found in approximately 80% of tumors, the Merkel cell polyomavirus (MCV) could play a key etiologic role. MCC usually develop on chronically sun-damaged skin. The most common sites of presentation are the head and neck region and extremities, followed by the trunk and oral and genital mucosa. Clinically it can range from erythematous plaques to erythematous or red, sometimes violaceous, sharply demarcated nodules with a smooth and shiny surface (Figure 34.1a, b). However, in the majority of cases MCC are "cherry red" in color, that is to say strikingly deep cherry red, a color spectrum ranging from dark red to violaceous, which helps to distinguish MCC from other red nodules such as Basal cell Carcinoma (BCC) and squamous cell carcinoma (SCC), which tend to be more pink (Figure 34.2a, b). Often they appeared opalescent. Tumor growth is usually very rapid. The most important clinical features of MCC are summarized under the acronym AEIOU: *a*symptomatic, rapid *e*xpansion, *i*mmunosuppression, *o*lder patient and located on *U*V-damaged skin.

DERMOSCOPY

Polymorphous vessels, which are defined as any combination of two or more different vascular structures, are the most important dermatoscopic criterion in MCC (Figure 34.3a, b).

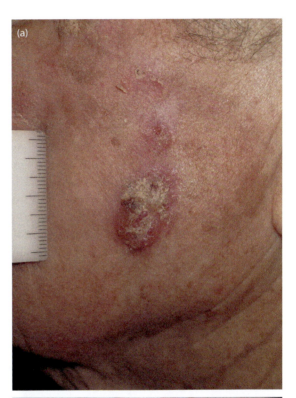

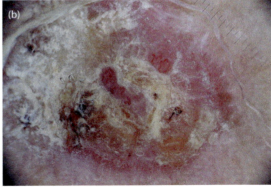

Figure 34.1 (a) A rare case of MCC characterized by a red nodule, a flat area with reddish background and hyperkeratosis. (b) Dermoscopy image shows the presence of polymorphous not-focused vessels.

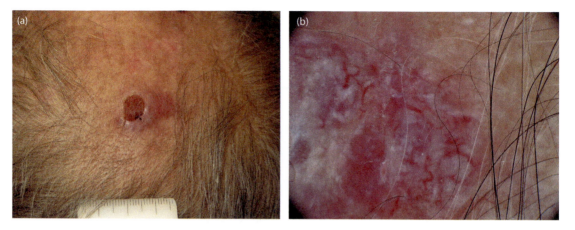

Figure 34.2 (a) Clinical view reveals a red nodule with reddish background on a scalp. (b) Dermoscopy image shows the presence of linear irregular vessels and milky red areas.

Linear, irregular not-focused vessels are most frequently found; they are linear and have irregular shapes, sizes and distribution, and are not in focus because vessels in MCC are deep intratumoral structures. Also dotted, glomerular and arborizing vessels can be observed in MCC: dotted vessels appear as adjacent tiny red dots, and glomerular vessels are a variation of dotted vessels, appearing as larger dots arranged in clusters similar to renal glomeruli. Arborizing vessels are defined as having a large-diameter stem vessel with finer irregular branches. Arborizing vessels that we observed in MCC appear to be located deeper within the tumor than BCC vessels and consequently are slightly out-of-focus and pink in color. Although BCC may be a diagnostic consideration in the MCC cases with arborizing vessels, the presence of other vascular patterns suggests a different pathology. Often MCC shows a reddish background. Furthermore, milky-red areas and white structureless areas can be present (Figure 34.4a, b). MCC vascular features are often also seen in amelanotic melanoma, but MCC has no tumor pigmentation or blue-white veil, which are common in melanoma. Glomerular vessels are common in Bowen's disease, which always shows a scaly surface, while hyperkeratosis generally is absent in MCC. Although no

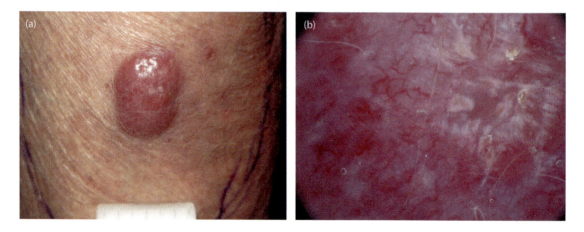

Figure 34.3 (a) Clinical view reveals a red nodule on the lower leg. (b) Dermoscopy image shows the presence of arborizing and linear irregular vessels along with crystalline structures.

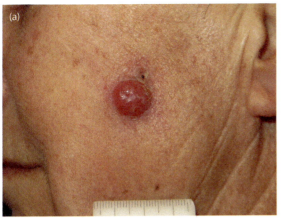 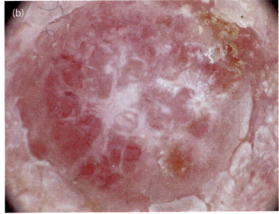

Figure 34.4 (a) Clinical image of a Merkel cell carcinoma arising on the left cheek of a 78-year-old woman. (b) Dermoscopy revealed milky red areas and irregular linear vessels.

specific dermatoscopic patterns have been found in MCC, the general rule still applies that every tumor exhibiting polymorphous vessels and/or milky-red areas should be excised, given that such patterns occur particularly often in malignant cutaneous tumors.[1–7]

REFERENCES

1. Deinlein T, Richtig G, Schwab C, Scarfi F, Arzberger E, Wolf I, Hofmann-Wellenhof R, Zalaudek I. The use of dermatoscopy in diagnosis and therapy of nonmelanocytic skin cancer. *J Dtsch Dermatol Ges*. 2016;**14**(2):144–51.
2. Lallas A, Moscarella E, Argenziano G, Longo C, Apalla Z, Ferrara G, Piana S, Rosato S, Zalaudek I. Dermoscopy of uncommon skin tumours. *Australas J Dermatol*. 2014;**55**(1):53–62.
3. Longo C, Benati E, Borsari S, Bombonato C, Pampena R, Moscarella E, Piana S, Pellacani G. Merkel cell carcinoma: Morphologic aspects on reflectance confocal microscopy. *J Eur Acad Dermatol Venereol*. 2017;**31**(11):e480–1.
4. Dalle S, Parmentier L, Moscarella E, Phan A, Argenziano G, Thomas L. Dermoscopy of Merkel cell carcinoma. *Dermatology*. 2012;**224**:140–4.
5. Jalilian C, Chamberlain AJ, Haskett M et al. Clinical and dermoscopic characteristics of Merkel cell carcinoma. *Br J Dermatol*. 2013;**169**:294–7.
6. Harting MS, Ludgate MW, Fullen DR et al. Dermatoscopic vascular patterns in cutaneous Merkel cell carcinoma. *J Am Acad Dermatol*. 2012;**66**:923–7.
7. Heath M, Jaimes N, Lemos B et al. Clinical characteristics of Merkel cell carcinoma at diagnosis in 195 patients: The AEIOU features. *J Am Acad Dermatol*. 2008;**58**:375–81.

35 Kaposi's sarcoma

Elisa Benati

INTRODUCTION

Kaposi's sarcoma (KS) is a vascular neoplasm first described by Kaposi in 1872. It can be divided into four clinical groups: classic, epidemic (associated with acquired immune deficiency syndrome [AIDS]), iatrogenic (in patients with immunosuppression) and endemic (African). Classic KS shows a predilection for elderly men (males to females, 10–15:1), and is more frequently found in people from Eastern Europe and the Mediterranean. The skin is the most common site, but internal organs may also be affected. In patients with classic KS, the vascular tumors are most commonly located on the lower extremities, especially the ankles and feet, whereas in people with AIDS-associated KS, the trunk is often involved (Figure 35.1a, b). Histologically, Kaposi's sarcoma is a vascular tumor characterized by a proliferation of spindle cells and endothelial cells to form closely arranged slit-like vascular spaces. KS lesions typically evolve through various stages as patches, plaques and nodules, and clinical lesions of different stages can often be seen in a single patient.

DERMOSCOPY

The most frequent dermoscopic patterns in Kaposi's sarcoma are bluish-reddish coloration, the "rainbow pattern" and scaly surface (Figures 35.2 through 35.4). Dermoscopy shows

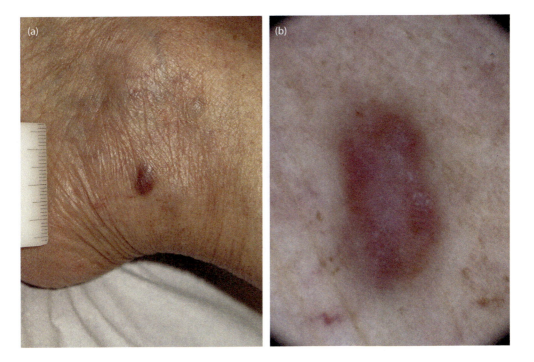

Figure 35.1 (a) Clinical view reveals a red nodule on the lower leg of a 75-year-old woman. (b) Dermoscopy image shows the presence of homogenous structureless whitish-red areas with scales.

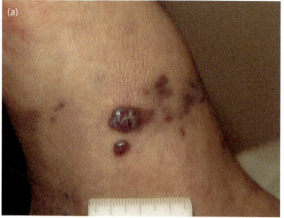
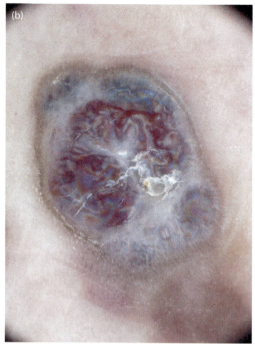

Figure 35.2 (a) Clinical image of a Kaposi's sarcoma arising on the foot of a 75-year-old man. He presented numerous dark nodules on his lower limbs and feet. (b) Dermoscopy revealed bluish-reddish coloration and the "rainbow pattern" under polarized dermoscopy.

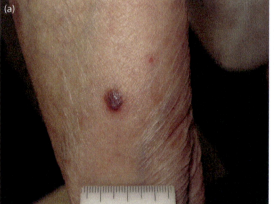
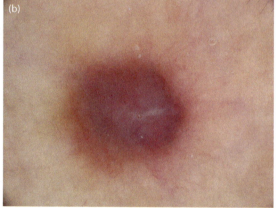

Figure 35.3 (a) Clinical view reveals a red nodule with reddish background on the arm of an 84-year-old woman. (b) Dermoscopy image shows the presence of white-reddish structureless areas, which reflect the vascular nature of Kaposi's sarcoma.

a bluish-reddish coloration, which reflects the vascular nature of Kaposi's sarcoma; a scaly surface, which could partly be a result of eczematous changes developing in some Kaposi's sarcoma lesions; and small brown globules and areas showing the distinctive multicolored "rainbow pattern" on polarized light dermoscopy. This dermoscopic feature, a multicolored "rainbow pattern," is highly specific but not sensitive for the diagnosis of KS, and it is possible

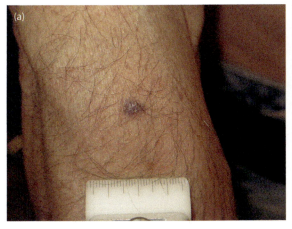
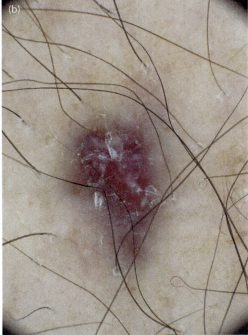

Figure 35.4 (a) A single lesion of the arm characterized by a red nodule with scales. (b) Dermoscopy image shows the presence of bluish-reddish coloration, the "rainbow pattern" and scaly surface.

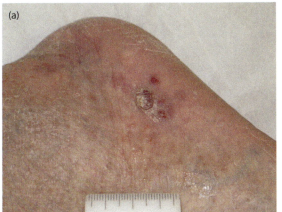
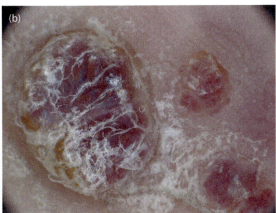

Figure 35.5 (a) Clinical view reveals red nodules on the foot of a 67-year-old man. (b) Dermoscopy image shows the presence of bluish-reddish background, the "rainbow pattern" and hyperkeratosis.

that non-KS lesions may produce the rainbow pattern under dermoscopy. In certain instances, this dermoscopic feature may reflect the richness of the vascular network of the skin lesion (Figures 35.5a, b and 35.6a, b). The "rainbow pattern" does not correspond to any concrete morphological structure on histology. It may rather represent an optical effect secondary to the interaction of light with the vascular structure of the tumor (Figure 35.7a, b).[1–3]

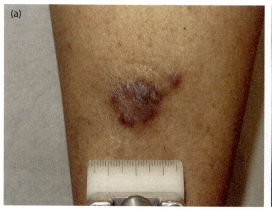
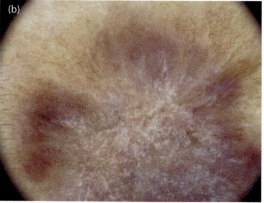

Figure 35.6 (a) Clinical image of a Kaposi's sarcoma arising on the leg of a 72-year-old woman. (b) Dermoscopy revealed white-reddish coloration (a); small brown globules were visualized in a few places (b); and the "rainbow pattern" was seen under polarized dermoscopy.

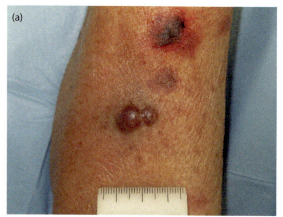
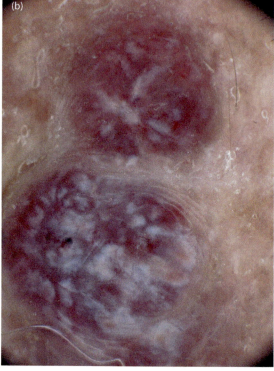

Figure 35.7 (a) Clinical image shows two violaceous nodules on the arm of a 76-year-old woman. (b) Dermoscopy revealed white-reddish coloration, and the "rainbow pattern" was seen under polarized dermoscopy.

REFERENCES

1. Cheng ST, Ke CL, Lee CH, Wu CS, Chen GS, Hu SC. Rainbow pattern in Kaposi's sarcoma under polarized dermoscopy: A dermoscopic pathological study. *Br J Dermatol*. 2009;**160**(4):801–9.
2. Hu SC, Ke CL, Lee CH, Wu CS, Chen GS, Cheng ST. Dermoscopy of Kaposi's sarcoma: Areas exhibiting the multicoloured "rainbow pattern". *J Eur Acad Dermatol Venereol*. 2009;**23**(10):1128–32.
3. Vázquez-López F, García-García B, Rajadhyaksha M, Marghoob AA. Dermoscopic rainbow pattern in non-Kaposi sarcoma lesions. *Br J Dermatol*. 2009;**161**(2):474–5.

36 Angiosarcoma

Elisa Benati

INTRODUCTION

Cutaneous angiosarcoma (AS) is a very rare tumor of endothelial origin characterized by a frequently aggressive clinical course and high metastatic potential. Predominantly affecting men, AS typically manifests after the age of 50 years. Cutaneous angiosarcomas are most common in the head and neck region. AS is considered to be the skin tumor with the poorest prognosis, with a 5-year survival rate of as low as 12%–20%. Cutaneous AS is divided into four clinical subtypes: sporadic angiosarcoma (AS) of the scalp and face; lymphedema-associated AS (LAS) arising typically in the context of Stewart–Treves syndrome; radiation-induced angiosarcoma (RIA) arising in previously

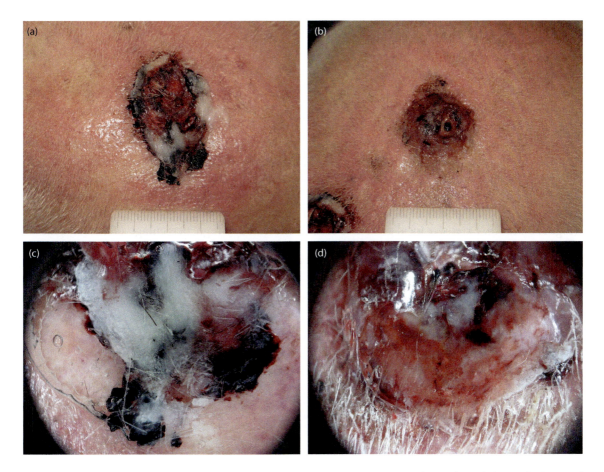

Figure 36.1 Angiosarcoma of the scalp. (a, b) Clinically it appears as an elevated, nodular and ulcerated lesion on the scalp. (c, d) Dermoscopy revealed structureless milky and red areas, scales and crusts.

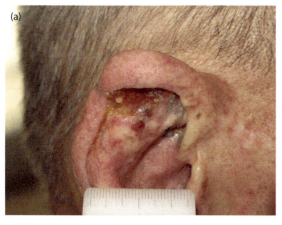 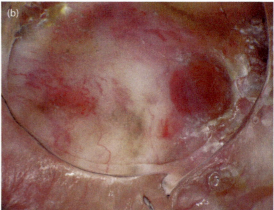

Figure 36.2 (a) Clinical view reveals an ulcerated area of the ear with a red nodule below. (b) Dermoscopy image shows the presence of polymorphous irregular vessels and structureless, red to violaceous areas that are intermingled with small yellow globular structures.

irradiated skin areas; and the recently described, very aggressive epithelioid subtype.

Clinically, early AS lesions develop as ill-defined violaceous to bluish areas with an indurated border. Angiosarcomas may present as hematoma-like macules, erythemato-violaceous plaques or nodules with poor demarcation from the surrounding tissue, thus mimicking lymphoma, hematoma or inflammatory dermatoses. Initial findings may also include erythema and subtle edema. The diagnosis of AS is often suspected at advanced stages when lesions become elevated or nodular and occasionally ulcerated (Figure 36.1a–d). Extensive local growth is common, and margins are difficult to define surgically. In approximately half of the patients the disease manifests with multiple separate foci. RIA and LAS tend to present as reddish to purple plaques with ill-defined borders.

ASs arising in chronic lymphedema of the extremities (Stewart–Treves syndrome) clinically are characterized by confluent erythemato-violaceous nodules or papules in the lymphedema-affected region of the extremity. Rarely angiosarcomas occur following radiation therapy, with reported latency periods between 3 and 10 years. Most commonly women are affected after radiation therapy for breast cancer.

DERMOSCOPY

AS typically exhibits structureless, red to violaceous or bluish areas that are intermingled with small yellow globular structures (Figure 36.2a, b). It is characterized by combinations of the typical colors of vascular tumors, namely, red, purple and blue (Figure 36.3a–f). Oiso et al. found a color gradation within ASs. They were able to show that different colors on dermatoscopy indicated a high percentage of tumor cells on histology. Another study described pink-violet steam-like areas as an important dermatoscopic feature to characterize AS. Vascular structures such as vessels or lacunae were not a dermatoscopic feature of AS, which might facilitate its differentiation from other vascular tumors such as hemangioma or angiokeratoma. By contrast, RIA dermatoscopically exhibits more homogenous, structureless, whitish-pink areas with increased color intensity at the periphery (Figure 36.4a, b). Early AS may resemble various inflammatory diseases, vascular tumors and amelanotic melanoma.[1–5]

ANGIOSARCOMA

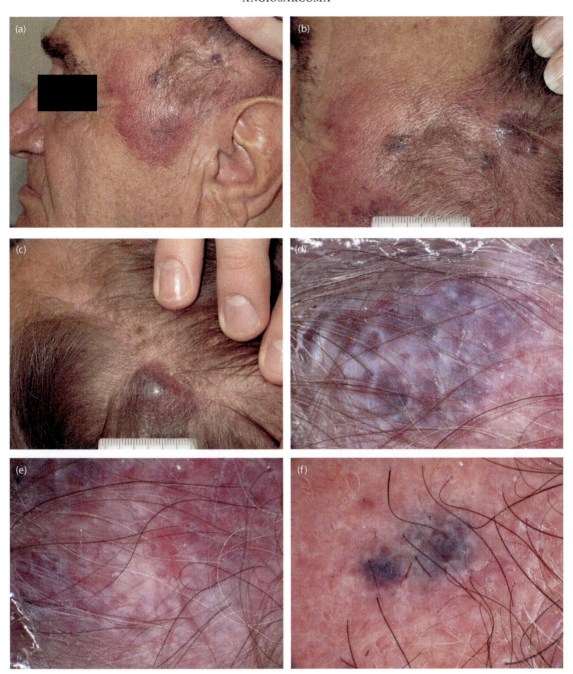

Figure 36.3 (a–c) Clinical view reveals red nodules on an erythematous flat lesion on the face and scalp. (d–f) Dermoscopy image shows the presence of structureless, red to violaceous or bluish areas.

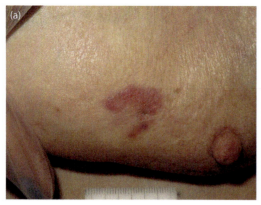
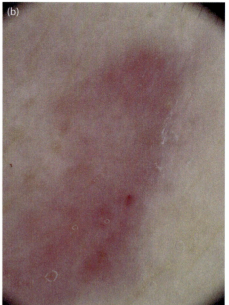

Figure 36.4 (a) A rare case of radiation-induced angiosarcoma (RIA) characterized by a flat area with a reddish background. (b) Dermatoscopically RIA exhibits homogenous, structureless, whitish-pink areas with increased color intensity at the periphery.

REFERENCES

1. Deinlein T, Richtig G, Schwab C, Scarfi F, Arzberger E, Wolf I, Hofmann-Wellenhof R, Zalaudek I. The use of dermatoscopy in diagnosis and therapy of nonmelanocytic skin cancer. *J Dtsch Dermatol Ges*. 2016;**14**(2):144–51.
2. Lallas A, Moscarella E, Argenziano G, Longo C, Apalla Z, Ferrara G, Piana S, Rosato S, Zalaudek I. Dermoscopy of uncommon skin tumours. *Australas J Dermatol*. 2014;**55**(1):53–62.
3. Kohlmeyer J, Steimle-Grauer SA, Hein R. Cutaneous sarcomas. *J Dtsch Dermatol Ges*. 2017;**15**(6):630–48.
4. Shustef E, Kazlouskaya V, Prieto VG, Ivan D, Aung PP. Cutaneous angiosarcoma: A current update. *J Clin Pathol*. 2017;**70**(11):917–25.
5. Oiso N, Matsuda H, Kawada A. Various colour gradations as a dermatoscopic feature of cutaneous angiosarcoma of the scalp. *Australas J Dermatol*. 2013;**54**(1):36–8.

37 Retiform hemangioendothelioma

Elisa Benati

INTRODUCTION

Hemangioendothelioma is a term encompassing neoplasms with an intermediate biological behavior between benign hemangiomas and angiosarcomas. Retiform hemangioendothelioma (RH) is an infrequently encountered vascular neoplasm of borderline malignancy that was originally classified as a distinct type of low-grade cutaneous angiosarcoma (CA). Histopathologically, the vascular channels of RH resemble the rete testis (retiform), while the term *hemangioendothelioma* reflects its putative borderline malignancy, as opposed to the benign angioma and the malignant angiosarcoma. Clinically, RH typically develops as a solitary, gradually enlarging exophytic mass, nodule or plaque, most often on the lower limbs, upper limbs and trunk (Figure 37.1a). The tumor shows a predilection for young to middle-aged adults (mean age 36 years) and females. A case of RH presenting with multiple lesions on the limbs and trunk has also been described. Surgical excision with tumor-free margins is the treatment of choice for RH, but the tumor is associated with a high rate of local recurrence (50%), regional lymph node metastasis was reported in a single patient, while no distant metastases have been reported to date.

DERMOSCOPY

Dermoscopy of RH reveals a pinkish color, which is also known to characterize amelanotic melanoma, Kaposi's sarcoma and cutaneous angiosarcoma and, effectively, cannot be considered as predictive of a specific diagnosis. However, since it has been only described in the context of malignant tumors, the detection

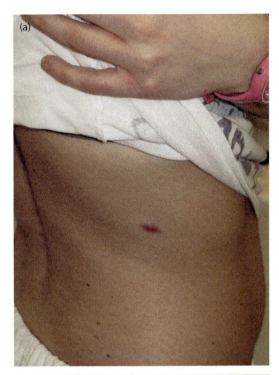

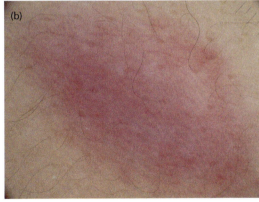

Figure 37.1 (a) Clinical examination revealed a well-defined, asymptomatic, rapidly enlarging, infiltrated, red nodule. (b) Dermoscopically, the tumor exhibited a pinkish background color and few dotted and linear vessels.

of pinkish (milky red) color led us to avoid misinterpretation of the tumor as benign and prompted us to perform a biopsy (Figure 37.1b). Undoubtedly, dermoscopic findings should always be integrated with clinical information; in fact the detection of pinkish color on dermoscopy of nodular lesions is suggestive of malignancy and should warrant excision.[1-7]

REFERENCES

1. Mota A, Argenziano G, Zalaudek I et al. Clinical, dermoscopic and histopathologic findings of retiform hemangioendothelioma. *Dermatol Pract Concept*. 2013;**3**(4):11-4.
2. Requena L, Kutzner H. Hemangioendothelioma. *Semin Diagn Pathol*. 2013;**30**(1):29-44.
3. Calonje E, Fletcher CD, Wilson-Jones E, Rosai J. Retiform hemangioendothelioma. A distinctive form of low-grade angiosarcoma delineated in a series of 15 cases. *Am J Surg Pathol*. 1994;**18**(2):115-25.
4. Duke D, Dvorak A, Harris TJ, Cohen LM. Multiple retiform hemangioendotheliomas. A low-grade angiosarcoma. *Am J Dermatopathol*. 1996;**18**(6):606-10.
5. Bhutoria B, Konar A, Chakrabartis S, Das S. Retiform hemangioendothelioma with lymph node metastasis: A rare entity. *Indian J Dermatol Venereol Leprol*. 2009;**75**(1):60-2.
6. Zalaudek I, Kreusch J, Giacomel J et al. How to diagnose non-pigmented skin tumors: A review of vascular structures seen with dermoscopy: Part 1. Melanocytic skin tumors. *J Am Acad Dermatol*. 2010;**63**(3):361-784.
7. Zalaudek I, Gomez-Moyano E, Landi C et al. Clinical, dermoscopic and histopathological features of spontaneous scalp or face and radiotherapy-induced angiosarcoma. *Australas J Dermatol*. 2013;**54**(3):201-7.

Index

A
Acquired immune deficiency syndrome (AIDS), 139
Acral melanoma (AM), 54–55
Adenosine 3,5′ monophosphate (AMP), 35
AEIOU, 135
AFX, *see* Atypical fibroxanthoma
AIDS, *see* Acquired immune deficiency syndrome
AM, *see* Acral melanoma
Amelanotic
  and partially ulcerated papule, 26
  and ulcerated nodule, 25
  melanoma, 53
  trichoepithelioma, 65
AMP, *see* Adenosine 3,5′ monophosphate
Angiosarcoma (AS), 143; *see also* Cutaneous angiosarcoma
  cutaneous, 147
  dermoscopy, 144
  radiation-induced, 143, 146
  red nodules on erythematous flat lesion on face and scalp, 145
  of scalp, 143
  ulcerated area of ear with red nodule, 144
Animal-type melanoma (ATM), 39
  blue-black nodule on upper back, 40
  brown-black nodule on arm, 39
  dermoscopy, 40
  satellite lesions, 39
AS, *see* Angiosarcoma
ASTs, *see* Atypical Spitz tumors
ATM, *see* Animal-type melanoma
Atypical fibroxanthoma (AFX), 127
  clinical image of, 127
  dermoscopy, 127, 129
  EFG rule, 127
  red nodule of cheek, 129
  red nodule on photo-damaged scalp, 128
  red nodule with scales of ear, 128
  red plaque on nose, 128
Atypical Spitz tumors (ASTs), 25
  amelanotic and partially ulcerated papule, 26
  amelanotic and ulcerated nodule, 25
  dermoscopy, 25, 27
  plaque on right ankle, 26
  red exophytic papule, 26
  taxonomy, 25
Autosomal dominant inheritance, genetic syndromes with, 101

B
Balloon cell malignant melanoma (BCMM), 47
  dermoscopy, 47–48
  erythematous, 47
  erythematous nodule, 48
Balloon melanoma cells (BMCs), 47
Basal cell carcinoma (BCC), 7, 11, 61, 63, 68, 70, 93, 101, 135; *see also* Nevoid basal cell carcinoma syndrome
  nonsyndromic and syndromic, 3
Basosquamous carcinoma, 11
  dermoscopy, 12–13
  ulcerated plaque, 11, 12, 13
BCMM, *see* Balloon cell malignant melanoma
Benign adnexal lesions, 93
BHDS, *see* Birt–Hogg–Dubè syndrome
Birt–Hogg–Dubè syndrome (BHDS), 85–86
Blue-black nodule on upper back, 40
Blue nodule
  on foot dorsum, 35
  on scalp, 36
BMCs, *see* Balloon melanoma cells
Brooke–Spiegler syndrome, 63, 101, 105
Brown
  -black nodule on arm, 39
  lesion with depigmented halo, 30
  -pinkish well-defined macule, 31

C
CA, *see* Cutaneous angiosarcoma
Calcifying epithelioma of Malherbe, *see* Pilomatrixoma
Carcinoma, syringomatous, 112
Carney complex, 35
Clear cell
  hidradenoma, *see* Nodular hidradenoma
  myoepithelioma, *see* Nodular hidradenoma
Crown vessels, 89
Cutaneous angiosarcoma (CA), 147
Cutaneous spindle cell tumors, malignant, 19; *see also* Sarcomatoid squamous cell carcinoma
Cutaneous tumors, 90
Cylindroma, 101, 102; *see also* Spiradenoma
  dermoscopy, 101
  multiple, 103
Cylindromatosis, familial, 101

D

Dark brown nodule on right arm, 44
Depigmented halo, lesion with, 30
Dermatofibrosarcoma of Darier and Ferrand, see Dermatofibrosarcoma protuberans
Dermatofibrosarcoma protuberans (DFSP), 123
   clinical image of, 123
   dermoscopy, 124–125
   red nodule, 124
Desmoplastic giant congenital melanocytic nevus (DGCN), 32; see also Desmoplastic nevus
Desmoplastic melanoma (DM), 49
   dermoscopy, 50–51
   diagnosis, 49
   pinkish nodule on forehead, 49
   well-defined nodule on nose, 50
Desmoplastic nevus, 31
   brown-pinkish well-defined macule, 31
   dermoscopy, 32
   pink papule with brown portion at periphery, 32
   well-defined nodule with translucent surface, 31
Desmoplastic trichoepithelioma (DTE), 67
   dermoscopy, 68
   with plaque-like appearance, 67
DFSP, see Dermatofibrosarcoma protuberans
DGCN, see Desmoplastic giant congenital melanocytic nevus
DM, see Desmoplastic melanoma
DTE, see Desmoplastic trichoepithelioma

E

Eccrine acrospiroma, see Nodular hidradenoma
Eccrine poroma, 115, 116, 117; see also Porocarcinoma
   dermoscopy, 115, 118
Eccrine sweat gland adenoma, see Nodular hidradenoma
EFG rule, 127
Epithelioma of Malherbe, calcifying, see Pilomatrixoma
Erythematous, 47
   flat lesion on face and scalp, 145
   nodule, 48
Exophytic
   nodular lesion, 93
   papule, red, 26

F

Familial cylindromatosis, 101
FeP, see Fibroepithelioma of pinkus
FFs, see Fibrofolliculomas
Fibroepithelioma of pinkus (FeP), 7
   dermoscopy, 7–8
   lesion, 7, 8
   papule, 8
Fibrofolliculomas (FFs), 85
   dermoscopy, 86
   multiple facial papules, 85, 86
Flesh-colored papule on left eyebrow, 61
Follicular keratosis, inverted, 73

G

Genetic syndromes with autosomal dominant inheritance, 101
Gorlin–Goltz syndrome (GS), 3; see also Nevoid basal cell carcinoma syndrome
GS, see Gorlin–Goltz syndrome

H

Halo reaction, 29
Halo Spitz nevus, 29
   brown lesion with depigmented halo, 30
   dermoscopy, 30
   well-defined papule, 29
Hemangioendothelioma, 147
Hidradenoma
   clear cell, see Nodular hidradenoma
   solid-cystic, see Nodular hidradenoma
HPV, see Human papillomavirus
Human papillomavirus (HPV), 15

I

Infundibuloma, see Tumors of follicular infundibulum
Inverted follicular keratosis, 73

K

Kaposi's sarcoma (KS), 139
   dermoscopy, 139
   on foot, 140, 141
   on leg, 142
   red nodule on lower leg, 139
   red nodule with reddish background on arm, 140
   red nodule with scales, 141
   violaceous nodules on arm, 142
Keratosis, inverted follicular, 73
KS, see Kaposi's sarcoma

L

LAS, see Lymphedema-associated AS
Lentigo maligna melanoma (LMM), 50
Lesions
   benign adnexal, 93
   with depigmented halo, 30
   satellite, 39
Linear irregular vessels and milky red areas, 136

LMM, *see* Lentigo maligna melanoma
Lymphedema-associated AS (LAS), 143

M
Macule, brown-pinkish well-defined, 31
Malignant cutaneous; *see also* Sarcomatoid squamous cell carcinoma
   spindle cell tumors, 19
   tumors, 90
Malignant fibrous histiocytoma (MFH), 127, 131
MCC, *see* Merkel cell carcinoma
MCV, *see* Merkel cell polyomavirus
mDM, *see* Mixed DM
Melanoma
   amelanotic, 53
   nail, 56
   Nevoid, 43
   oral, 53
   primary cutaneous, 53
   sinonasal mucosal, 53
   of special site, 53
   vulvar, 53, 54
Melanosarcoma, 39
Merkel cell carcinoma (MCC), 135
   dermoscopy, 135–137
   on left cheek, 137
   linear irregular vessels and milky red areas, 136
   red nodule, 135, 136
Merkel cell polyomavirus (MCV), 135
MFH, *see* Malignant fibrous histiocytoma
Mixed DM (mDM), 50; *see also* Desmoplastic melanoma
Mucosal melanomas, 53
Muir–Torre syndrome, 89
Multicolored plaque, 44
Multiple facial papules, 85, 86
Myoepithelioma, clear cell, *see* Nodular hidradenoma

N
Nail melanoma, 56
NBCCS, *see* Nevoid basal cell carcinoma syndrome
NeM, *see* Nevoid melanoma
Nevoid basal cell carcinoma syndrome (NBCCS), 3
   dermoscopy, 4–5
   lesion, 4
   palmar pits, 5
   translucent papule, 4
Nevoid melanoma (NeM), 43
   dark brown nodule on right arm, 44
   dermoscopy, 43
   multicolored plaque, 44
   skin-colored papillomatous plaque, 43

Nodular hidradenoma, 97
   dermoscopy, 98–99
   nonpigmented cases of, 97
   pigmented cases of, 98
Nodular lesion, exophytic, 93
Nodule; *see also* Kaposi's sarcoma; Nodular hidradenoma
   amelanotic ulcerated, 25
   blue, 35, 36
   blue-black, 40
   brown-black, 39
   dark brown, 44
   on erythematous flat lesion, 145
   erythematous, 48
   heavily pigmented, 37
   on forehead, 49
   on lower leg, 139
   on nose, 50
   pinkish, 49
   red, 124, 128, 129
   ulcerated area of ear with, 144
   violaeous, 142
   with reddish background, 140
   with scales, 128, 141
   with translucent surface, 31

O
OMIM, *see* Online Mendelian Inheritance in Man
Online Mendelian Inheritance in Man (OMIM), 63, 89, 101
Oral florid papillomatosis, 15; *see also* Verrucous carcinoma
OS, *see* Overall survival
Overall survival (OS), 50

P
Paget's disease, 107
   dermoscopy, 107
   extramammary, 107, 109
   mammary, 108
Palmar pits, 5
Papules
   facial, 85, 86
   on eyebrow, 61
   pink with brown at periphery, 32
   translucent, 4
   flesh-colored papule, 61
   amelanotic and partially ulcerated, 26
   on shoulder, well-defined, 29
   red exophytic, 26
   multiple facial, 85, 86
PAS, *see* Periodic acid–Schiff
pDM, *see* Pure DM
PEM, *see* Pigmented epithelioid melanocytoma
Periodic acid–Schiff (PAS), 77, 105

Pigmented epithelioid melanocytoma (PEM), 35, 39
    blue nodule on foot dorsum, 35
    blue nodule on scalp, 36
    dermoscopy, 37
    heavily pigmented nodule, 37
Pigmented nodule on back, 37
Pilomatricoma, *see* Pilomatrixoma
Pilomatrixoma, 81
    dermoscopy, 83
Pinkish nodule on forehead, 49
Pink papule with brown portion at periphery, 32
Plaque
    in vertex of scalp, 94
    multicolored, 44
    on ankle, 26
    skin-colored papillomatous, 43
    ulcerated, 11, 12, 13
Pleomorphic undifferentiated sarcoma, *see* Malignant fibrous histiocytoma
Porocarcinoma, 115, 117; *see also* Eccrine poroma
Primary cutaneous melanoma, 53
Pure DM (pDM), 50; *see also* Desmoplastic melanoma

R
R1α, *see* Regulatory subunit 1α
Radiation-induced angiosarcoma (RIA), 143, 146
Red exophytic papule, 26
Red nodule, 124, 135, 136
    of cheek, 129
    on photo-damaged scalp, 128
    on lower leg, 139
    reddish background on arm, 140
    with scales, 128, 141
    on erythematous flat lesion on face and scalp, 145
Red plaque on nose, 128
Regulatory subunit 1α (R1α), 35
Retiform hemangioendothelioma (RH), 147
    dermoscopy, 147–148
RH, *see* Retiform hemangioendothelioma
RIA, *see* Radiation-induced angiosarcoma

S
Sarcomatoid squamous cell carcinoma (SSCC), 19
    dermoscopy, 20
    on neck, 19
    on scalp, 20
Satellite lesions, 39
Scalp nodule, 36
SCAP, *see* Syringocystadenoma papilliferum
SCC, *see* Squamous cell carcinoma
Sclerotic nevus, *see* Desmoplastic nevus
Sebaceous tumors, 89
    benign, 90, 91
    dermoscopy, 89, 91
    malignant cutaneous tumors, 90

Serpentine vessels, 51
Sinonasal mucosal melanoma, 53
Skin-colored papillomatous plaque, 43
Solid-cystic hidradenoma, *see* Nodular hidradenoma
Special site melanoma, 53
Spindle cell tumors, malignant cutaneous, 19; *see also* Sarcomatoid squamous cell carcinoma
Spiradenoma, 105; *see also* Cylindroma
Spitz nevus, 29
Squamous cell carcinoma (SCC), 11, 19, 93, 135
SSCC, *see* Sarcomatoid squamous cell carcinoma
Stewart–Treves syndrome, 144
Syringocystadenoma papilliferum (SCAP), 93
    dermoscopy, 94
    exophytic nodular lesion, 93
    globular structures with irregular vessels, 94
    plaque in vertex of scalp, 94
    verrucous yellowish lesion, 93
Syringoma, 111
    dermoscopy, 112–113
    multiple, 111
    syringomatous carcinoma, 112
Syringomatous carcinoma, 112

T
TDs, *see* Trichodiscomas
Translucent papule, 4
Trichoadenoma, 61
    dermoscopy, 62
    flesh-colored papule on left eyebrow, 61
Trichoblastoma, 69
    dermoscopy, 70–71
Trichodiscomas (TDs), 85–86
Trichoepithelioma, 63
    amelanotic, 65
    dermoscopy, 63
    located on face, 64
Tricholemmoma, 77
    dermoscopy, 78–79
    ulcerated nonpigmented nodule, 78
Tumors, cutaneous, 90
Tumors of follicular infundibulum, 73
    dermoscopy, 73–74
    inverted follicular keratosis, 73

U
Ulcerated
    area of ear with red nodule, 144
    nonpigmented nodule, 78
    plaque, 11, 12, 13
    papule, amelanotic and partially, 26
    amelanotic nodule, 25
Ultraviolet (UV), 49

V

VC, *see* Verrucous carcinoma
Verrucous carcinoma (VC), 15
  anogenital, 15
  dermoscopy, 16–17
  genital, 15
  locations of, 15
  palmoplantar, 15
  periungual, 16
  on right sole, 16
  yellowish lesion, 93

Violaeous nodules on arm, 142
Vulvar melanoma (VM), 53, 54
  dermoscopy, 55

W

Well-defined nodule; *see also* Nodule
  on nose, 50
  with translucent surface, 31
Well-defined papule on shoulder, 29

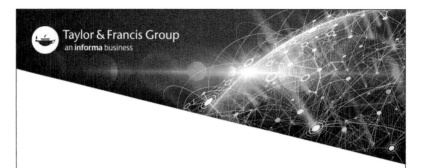